Empty Eating

Empty Eating

HOW TO STOP EATING HIGH-CALORIE, LOW-NUTRIENT FOOD

Chef Bill Collins

http://www.chefbillcollins.com https://www.facebook.com/
ChefBillCollins/ https://www.emptyeating.com
https://www.fibermega.com
https://www.facebook.com/fibermega/

ISBN-13: 9781535496421
ISBN-10: 1535496428

Disclaimer

This book is intended as a reference only, not as a medical manual. The information given is designed to help you make informed decisions about your health. It is not intended as a substitute for any treatment that your doctor may have prescribed. If you suspect that you have a medical problem, I urge you to seek competent medical help.

Mention of specific companies, organizations, or authorities in this book does not imply their endorsement by the author or publisher, nor does it imply that they endorse this book, its author, or the publisher.

Internet addresses and telephone numbers given in this book were accurate at the time of publication.

Dedication

This book is dedicated to some of my family members who are fighting diabetes, high blood pressure, and obesity.

I wrote it for my loved ones and for the millions of people who want to live a disease-free, healthy, and energetic lifestyle but don't know how to get started. My goal is to provide you with a pathway to a healthy life, free of disease.

I sincerely believe many illnesses can be abolished if we change our diets to high-nutrient, low-calorie food. As a chef who understands the impact of food on our bodies, I want to help you with your food and health challenges and choices.

Acknowledgments

Thank you to my family, friends, and mentors who have supported me throughout this project. I also appreciate Ms. Cora Wallace and her son, Shedric Wallace, my business associate and confidant.

Foreword

Congratulations! By choosing to read *Empty Eating*, you've taken the first and most important step toward improving your health. Someone said, "How a person thinks determines his or her reality." Therefore, the most powerful step in your journey to excellent health begins with changing your beliefs about what it means to live healthy.

My journey started years ago when a friend handed me a book on nutrition that dramatically changed my understanding of healthy eating. More than a decade later, I now work in close collaboration with Chef Bill Collins, spreading the truth of healthy eating through the Culinary Wellness Institute (CWI).

Although many health experts offer advice these days, Chef Bill Collins stands apart for two obvious reasons. First, Chef Bill Collins provides straight talk. Unlike many nutritionists and medical doctors who write books, he does not waste time on complicated medical theories. In *Empty Eating*, Chef Bill gets straight to the point—providing practical advice on how to improve your health.

Second, Chef Bill is a role model for the principles he teaches. For many years, before he discovered the benefit of nutrient-dense whole-plant food, Chef Bill consumed quite a few of the foods against which he now warns his readers. Back then, he was overweight, unhealthy, and on the verge of going on medication. As a fellow chef and wellness advocate, I watched Chef Bill Collins educate himself, change his eating habits, and restore his health. He knows what it takes to get and stay both lean and healthy.

As you read his book, Chef Bill will challenge your current thinking. He understands that better health begins with better thinking; in other words, "If you do what you've always done, you will get what you always got."

One of the most common challenges Chef Bill and I encounter with people new to healthful eating is something we call the "Bacon Paradox." People often say, "I want to improve my health, but I love bacon, and nobody is going to make me give it up." The truth is that most of us love the taste of bacon, ice cream, and potato chips—these foods are *designed* to be super tasty and addictive. More importantly, no one can make another person stop eating the foods he or she enjoys. That is not the goal of *Empty Eating*.

This book is mostly about learning to eat more of the foods that improve and support health. Unfortunately, many people have survived so long with unhealthful eating habits that they have forgotten what it feels like to be healthy. Cutting back on "empty calories" and eating more nutrient-dense foods is the key to better health. That includes having strength, energy, clear thoughts, radiant skin, less physical stress, an attractive body, and protection against disease. Since that's true, sign me up for that program. If most people understood what Chef Bill Collins is offering in this book, they would not hesitate to read and follow his wise advice. I recommend reading *Empty Eating* and letting the message soak in deeply. Then make a commitment to implement its principles gradually. After all, health is a journey!

Chef Shedric
The Healthful Chef
HealthfulChef.com

Contents

Introduction

Several decades ago, society faced certain illnesses called "diseases of the affluent"—so named because only rich people contracted them. These included conditions such as type 2 diabetes, asthma, coronary heart disease, obesity, hypertension, cancer, alcoholism, gout, and various allergies. These NCDs (noncommunicable diseases) were not transmitted by contact with someone who had the condition; instead, they resulted from poor health choices.

At one time, only the wealthy could afford to eat meat, dairy, and processed foods on a regular basis. Thanks to modern refrigeration and packaging systems, however, most people are now able to eat meat, dairy, and processed foods every day. This has become the nutritional norm in America.

Let's explore some vital information about the impact of this type of diet.

My family and I have faced some personal health challenges—ones that are all too common in today's society.

The other day, a good friend and I were discussing our behavioral challenges. He commented, "I am fighting off demons daily." He meant that no matter how disciplined his lifestyle appears, he fights the urge to indulge himself with pizza, chicken wings, or an all-American cheeseburger every day. He is not alone in that struggle.

When I share nutritional information, my family and friends sometimes aren't willing to accept the truth about various foods and their effects on our bodies. I can usually see a subtle disdain in their body language or facial expressions or hear it in their tone of voice. Some even become vocal to defend their positions. When this happens, I smile and move to another topic to avoid a debate.

Contrary to what some of us believe, science has proven how damaging certain lifestyle choices can be. Researchers have shown that people with type 2 diabetes who refuse to change their diet and exercise regimes have a high probability of contracting other diseases. Some of my family members have painfully illustrated this point.

If you want to learn how to lose weight and improve your health, you need to understand the concept of Empty Eating. Empty Eating is consuming high-calorie, low-nutrient food. Although the definition is short and straightforward, changing from that diet is not easy. Many people are addicted to these delicious but harmful foods. Dishes such as fried chicken, hamburgers, and pizza fit this description; in fact, most foods, except plant-based foods, fit into the "empty calorie" category. It is that simple.

Many of you who are reading this have made a conscious decision to improve your life by eating healthier foods. You may also have some other health problems, such as being overweight. Some dietary health issues may have encouraged you to consider a radical change, beginning with this book.

After you read this book and adopt its principles, your life will change for the better. That includes positive side effects such as losing weight, increasing energy, and feeling healthier.

By choosing to read this book, you are demonstrating that you *do* care for your body. The best way for you to be successful is to "just do it," so you can experience a much healthier lifestyle as soon as possible.

It will not be easy, but it will be worth it. My job is helping you transition to that rewarding new lifestyle, regardless of challenges you may face. I will help you break through the misinformation and misguided beliefs that hold many of us back.

If I can help you embrace a lifestyle built on plant-based food, you soon will see changes in your weight and will experience a greater sense of well-being.

I do not want to bore you with facts, but some are necessary for you to be convinced you are making the right decision. Together, we will look at the most recent information provided by researchers and scientists; much of this research comes from leading universities and research hospitals, who have published further findings on their websites. These reports will give you additional scientific data supporting the benefits of plant-based food. I have often wondered why the media doesn't make this the lead story on television newscasts and report it in documentaries. Incredible as it seems, the media has lied to us about healthy eating. Apparently, it isn't profitable for corporations to keep people healthy eating plant-based food.

For the principles in this book to work, you will have to make the specific changes outlined in these pages. Eventually, you will master a new lifestyle that will become as natural to you as waking up in the morning.

I strongly recommend surrounding yourself with a support group of individuals who share your passion for becoming a healthier person. Be sure to spend time with people who share the same goals.

Even as you make progress, you can also make some bad choices. If you do, don't beat yourself up. Just forgive yourself, and keep moving forward.

CHAPTER 1
What Is Empty Eating?

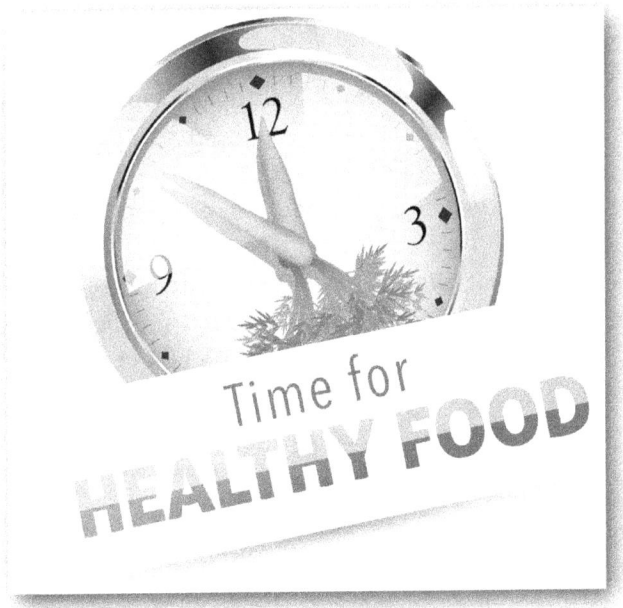

believe we all know someone who can eat a lot of food but not worry about gaining an ounce. Those of us who are health conscious also know someone who says, "I can get fat just thinking about food."

In reality, some people do appear to eat much less than others and still gain weight. Trying to lose weight is a battle. For many people, that battle is lost before it starts. Their subconscious minds tell them, "You don't want to do this! You'll have to sacrifice eating all the great-tasting food you love." Losing weight appears difficult or impossible; therefore, we give up before we start. I have often wondered, "Why is this happening?" With my years of experience, I have found there is not one cause but many.

Many experts in nutrition have difficulty explaining why some people can't lose weight. To clarify this issue, I am going to explain how to avoid the one thing I consider the biggest reason so many people fail to become healthy. A single issue contributes to significant weight gain and other debilitating health problems; doctors and scientists call this hidden danger Empty Eating.

The quality of your health depends on the type of food you consume. I intend to help you choose the healthiest food to maintain a healthy body. All low-calorie, high-nutrient food is good. High-calorie, low-nutrient food will lead your body toward poor health and multiple diseases.

Calories are not the only things our bodies get from food, as the body also needs the nutrients that food supplies. Healthy food consists of vitamins, minerals (the building blocks of proteins), and some healthy fats, as well as different types of carbohydrates and phytochemicals. You may be shocked to read this, but not all fats are harmful to your body. Some fatty acids, such as those in some fruits (avocados), nuts (such as walnuts), and seeds (like flax seeds) are very beneficial to our health.

Nutrient Density

We all agree that food provides a range of different nutrients. Some nutrients provide energy, while others are essential for growth and maintenance of the body.

Carbohydrates, protein, and fat are macronutrients that we need to eat daily. They provide our bodies with energy and the building blocks for growth and maintenance of health. Vitamins, minerals, and phytochemicals are micronutrients, which we need in only small amounts, but they are essential to keep us healthy.

According to the National Health and Research Council, "Water is defined as an essential nutrient because it is required in amounts that exceed the body's ability to produce it." According to the Harvard T. H. Chan School of Public Health, "Fiber is a type of carbohydrate that the body can't digest. Though most carbohydrates are broken down into sugar molecules, fiber cannot be broken down into sugar molecules, and instead, it passes through the body undigested. Fiber helps regulate the body's use of sugars, helping to keep hunger and blood sugar in check."

Water and fiber have no nutrients, but we can't live without them.

"Nutrient density" is the ratio of nutrients to calories in foods. It is an important concept to remember for health, especially for someone trying to lose weight. Nutrient density is, in short, the quantities of nutrients in a food compared to the calories in that food. This is important because the more calories food has, the more weight we gain; the more nutrients food has, the healthier that food is for the body. Foods high in calories but low in nutrients are not healthy. To put this in perspective, let's say you have a pound of broccoli clusters, which has approximately 154 calories. If you compare that to a pound of 90 percent lean ground beef, you'll find the meat has more than six times the calories of the broccoli.

On the other hand, micronutrients (such as vitamins, minerals, phytochemicals, and fiber) are just as important. These noncaloric nutrients do not produce energy as carbohydrates, fats, and proteins do.

When we compare how many nutrients a food item contains with how many calories it has, we see how different foods are. Some foods have a lot of calories but few nutrients, while others have plenty of nutrients but very few calories. Those foods with a lot of nutrients and not many calories are healthy—with an extra benefit of helping with weight loss. Nutritionists classify these as high-nutrient foods. Foods high in calories are not the best choice for maintaining good health, because they have so little nutrient value. I categorize many of these foods as "empty calories."

Speaking scientifically, according to the World Health Organization, nutrient profiling classifies and ranks foods by their nutritional composition to promote health and help prevent disease.[1] Hunter and Cason of Clemson University define nutrient density as "a measure of the nutrients provided per calorie of food, or the ratio of nutrients to calories (energy)."[2] This means empty calories are ones that are not accompanied by many nutrients. Food that is high in calories has a direct impact on weight gain. Macronutrients are required to maintain high energy levels, and micronutrients help maintain good health. It's hard to have a deficiency in macronutrients, although the correct balance is different in each person, and it takes a conscientious effort to achieve the optimal balance.

While we discuss the importance of nutrients and calories to our health, we must realize that not all calories are the same. According to fatsecret.com, a 1.5-ounce milk chocolate candy bar has 235 calories, and 100 grams (approximately 3.5 ounces) of cooked broccoli florets has 35 calories. (I've based these nutrition values on the USDA nutrient database.) I use this example because most people can relate to and visualize the amounts. My point is that all calories provide energy, but not all calories are equal. According to my friend Shedric Wallace, author of *The MicroNutrient Solution*, "Sugar will cause a spike in insulin, quickly turn to fat, provide no needed nutrients, and create long-term metabolic problems if consumed often." In contrast, the body digests broccoli slowly, without causing an insulin spike, and broccoli provides many valuable nutrients, helps cleanse the body by contributing fiber, and contributes to long-term health when eaten.

Many foods that contain empty calories have simple carbohydrates (sugars), ethanol (alcohols), and in some cases, fats (particularly solid fats, such as shortening, butter, and lard).[3]

Physical activity also contributes to weight loss. Exercise causes you to burn more calories. When you burn more calories, you can consume more calories daily without worrying about gaining weight. However, while exercise does cause you to burn more calories, this does not mean you have the green light to consume empty calories. Remember, not all calories are equal, and there is no way to maintain good health while eating empty calories. Also, you cannot exercise your way to good health without also eating high-nutrient food.

Overweight and obese people trying to lose weight are the most vulnerable to having health issues, because they frequently eat high-calorie, low-nutrient food more often than do food-conscious people. Food-savvy or nutritionally aware people know they need nutrients such as vitamins, minerals, and healthy fats to maintain a healthy body. Not eating healthy food daily may lead to certain diseases, including malnutrition.[4] If you are already on a limited diet (eating less and trying to lose weight) or you are counting calories, you should pay particular attention to the nutrients in the food you consume. If you are eating empty calories, you will probably suffer from one of the diseases and conditions caused by malnutrition.[5] This can lead to many complications; even if you lose weight, you will have lost it at the cost of your health.

Eating a variety of foods—such as vegetables, grains, nuts, seeds, and fruits—is essential to maintaining health, because the diversity allows you to get all the nutrients you need. It prevents chronic diseases, helps you lose weight, and helps strengthen the immune system so the body can fight against infections. To maintain good health, eat nutrients. The Academy of Nutrition and Dietetics recommends that you substitute legumes (beans and peas) for meats and dairy and swap whole wheat flour for white flour. Whole-food plant-based foods are the best way to eat if you want the most nutrients and the fewest calories.[6]

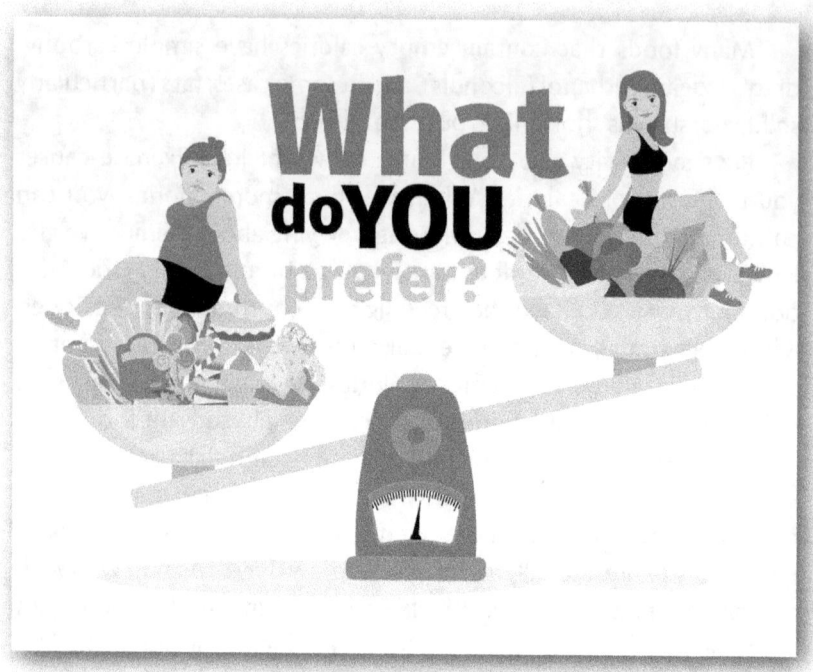

Quality versus Quantity

The result of consuming a large amount of food is usually consuming more calories. Overeating one type of food while neglecting others can lead to malnutrition. Malnutrition is a condition that results from not getting enough of a variety of nutrients (vitamins and minerals). You should not think a meal is healthy just because it is filling. Every meal should be balanced and should include the healthiest foods, such as whole grains, legumes, and leafy greens. If you eat food that is high in calories, such as meats, fast food, cheese, and fatty foods, you will have a tendency to eat more in order to get enough nutrients. Eating more of these foods will make you gain weight.

The number of calories you consume has a significant impact on weight. You may need to limit the number of calories you eat daily, depending on your weight.[7] People usually start to gain weight because they overeat empty calories. They usually eat much more than they actually need for good health and also maintain low levels of activity, if they have any activity at all.

I want to stress the importance of quality versus quantity and restate that overeating empty calories is a primary reason people get fat. High-calorie food, such as fast food, refined grains, fatty meats, and sweets are the main culprits. These foods, in addition to being high in calories, don't have enough nutrients and lead to health complications.

Portion sizes have created a lot of debate. The size of the portion you eat is as important as the foods you eat. Eating large meals two or three times per day is an option I consider harmful. Some believe the healthiest way to eat is to have several smaller meals in a day and make sure they are packed with nutrient-rich foods, such as vegetables, leafy greens, legumes, and whole grains. When trying to lose weight and achieve optimal health, it is important to eat as many nutrient-rich foods as possible and avoid eating high-calorie foods; this will ensure you are getting enough nutrients and calories. Eating multiple meals containing 300 to 400 calories each and consisting of high-nutrient foods is the most efficient way to have a healthy diet and maintain a healthy body weight. Eating like this will give you all the vitamins and minerals needed. I personally believe you—and only you—know what is best for you when it comes to the size of your meals; we are all different, and what works for me may not do the same for you. However, a nutritional plan is essential. Just remember you do not have to stuff yourself at every meal.

Nutrient-Dense versus Energy-Dense Foods

According to nutrition authorities such as the USDA, the WHO, and the Academy of Nutrition and Dietetics, foods can be divided into two categories: *nutrient-dense foods* and *energy-dense foods*. Nutrient-dense foods are high-nutrient, low-calorie foods containing more vitamins, minerals, phytochemicals, and fiber. Energy-dense foods are high-calorie foods with fewer nutrients than you'll find in nutrient-dense foods.[8] When you eat energy-dense foods, you're eating empty calories. Our daily caloric needs are the number of calories we should eat in a day. In contrast, the recommended amount of nutrients a person should eat in a day is our daily nutrient need. Table 1 shows how many calories in total (and the maximum number of empty calories) you should eat in a day, based on daily caloric and nutrient requirements.

Table 1. Daily empty-calorie allowance based on age (retrieved from choosemyplate.gov)

Age and gender	Estimated calories for those who are not physically active	
	Total daily calorie needs	Daily limit for empty calories
Children 2-3	1000 cal	135
Children 4-8 yrs	1200-1400 cal	120
Girls 9-13 yrs	1600 cal	120
Boys 9-13 yrs	1800 cal	160
Girls 14-18 yrs	1800 cal	160
Boys 14-18 yrs	2200 cal	265
Females 19-30 yrs	2000 cal	260
Males 19-30 yrs	2400 cal	330
Females 31-50 yrs	1800 cal	160
Males 31-50 yrs	2200 cal	265
Females 51+ yrs	1600 cal	120
Males 51+ yrs	2000 cal	260

How do you know which foods contain empty calories and which foods do not? Nutritionists and other food professionals know exactly how many calories and nutrients are in every food, but nonprofessionals are often unaware of the specific data for each kind of food; even though nutritional facts are on food labels, not everyone understands the information they are reading. Those of us who are trying to be healthy and lose weight should know a few basic facts about some foods to avoid and the reasons why.

Based on the number of calories in some ingredients used to make various foods, the nutritional facts will give you a general idea of what foods to avoid. Foods with ingredients such as shortening (animal fats, such as butter, lard, or beef fat), high amounts of sugar, or refined grains are all rich in calories but low in nutrients. Eating foods like these will contribute to weight gain and will starve your body of valuable nutrients. For an easy comparison, a female twenty-five years of age has a limit of 260 empty calories per day. That amounts to fewer than two ounces of a chocolate bar, milk, plain (Hershey Bar, Kiss, Nestle Bar) or fewer than two ounces of any kind of nuts, including peanuts (data obtained via USDA's site: http://www.supertracker. usda.gov). Anything more than that will contribute to weight gain, unless it is burned off by exercise.

Some foods generally considered high in calories and low in nutrients include the following:

- Most sweets, such as cake, cookies, candy, ice cream, and gelatin and other foods containing added sugars, including high-fructose corn syrup and commercial sweeteners
- Sweetened beverages, such as sodas, other soft drinks, fruit-flavored beverages, and sweetened fruit juices
- Solid fats, such as margarine or shortening, and other fats and oils considered low in healthy fatty acids
- Alcoholic beverages, such as beer, wine, spirits, and similar sweet drinks, such as liqueurs and cocktails
- Most fast foods, such as pizza, burgers, fries, and fried chicken
- Fatty meats, such as bacon and other meats that aren't as lean
- Refined grains, such as white flour and white rice

How one prepares food also has an effect on calories and nutrients. That means some cooking methods are not as healthy as others are and may lead to weight gain. If we consume food fried in oil or over-cooked, or if the cook adds sugar, the calorie count will increase. That changes the ratio of nutrients to calories. This means that if you eat a healthy, low-calorie, high-nutrient food such as vegetables, but you have it fried, it will not be as healthy as if it were steam-cooked. It's best to boil, steam, or bake food with little or no oils for more efficient nutrient absorption.

As much as possible, avoid these cooking practices:

- Deep-fat frying
- Baking with fats and skin
- Overcooking vegetables
- Adding sugars to desserts
- Using refined grains

Another method you can use to help you to lose weight is to start reading labels. Many commercial foods have added sugars. Baked goods using refined grains, commercial salads, and commercial pre-packaged meals often have many additives and additional sweeteners. Added sweeteners and additives sometimes make the food taste better, but the extra calories work against achieving optimal health.

By consuming high amounts of nutrient-dense food, you can eat as much as you like and maintain good health. In addition, you do not have to worry about counting or overconsuming calories. Most fruits and vegetables are nutrient-rich foods, so you should consume fruits and vegetables at every meal.

Dr. Joel Fuhrman based his Nutritarian food pyramid on the principles of high-nutrient eating.[9] The bottom of the pyramid represents vegetables and high-nutrient foods. Dr. Fuhrman believes you should avoid low-nutrient foods entirely or should eat them rarely and in small amounts; he says you should leave out empty calories altogether.

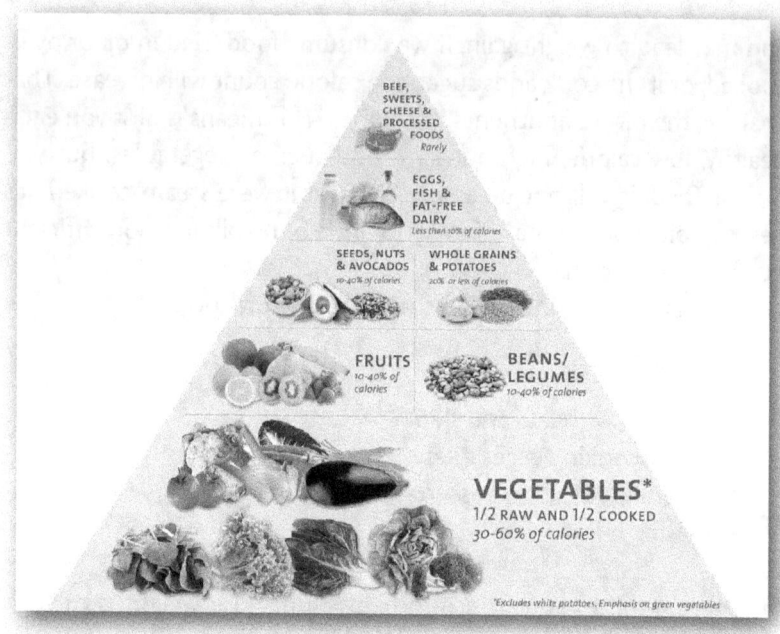

Figure 1. Dr. Fuhrman's Nutritarian food pyramid (www.drfuhrman.com)

An ideal meal contains as many nutrient-rich foods as possible, while at the same time avoiding calorie-dense foods, so you can eat as many nutrients as you want. Viewing the pyramid, you can see that you should consume leafy greens and most vegetables in larger amounts than other items with every meal. You should also eat beans and legumes daily, but they should be consumed in smaller quantities, and whole grains, nuts, and seeds should be eaten in even lower amounts. Nuts have valuable nutrients, but they also contain high amounts of fat. Overeating nuts can be counterproductive if you are trying to lower your weight. An ounce or two of nuts should be your maximum daily allowance.

I've based my daily diet on the principles of high-nutrient eating. The best diet is from vegetables, most of which are high-nutrient foods. You should avoid low-nutrient foods or eat it in small amounts and should avoid empty calories, such as sweets or soft drinks. This means your meals should be made up of whole plant–based food such as vegetables, greens, legumes, nuts, and seeds. If you eat animal foods, you should only have lean meats and fat-free dairy. You should consume these only in limited amounts. Avoid high-fat and high-sugar foods as much as possible. That means things you should avoid foods such as cheese, sweets, deep-fried foods and all refined as much as possible if you want to lose weight. [10]

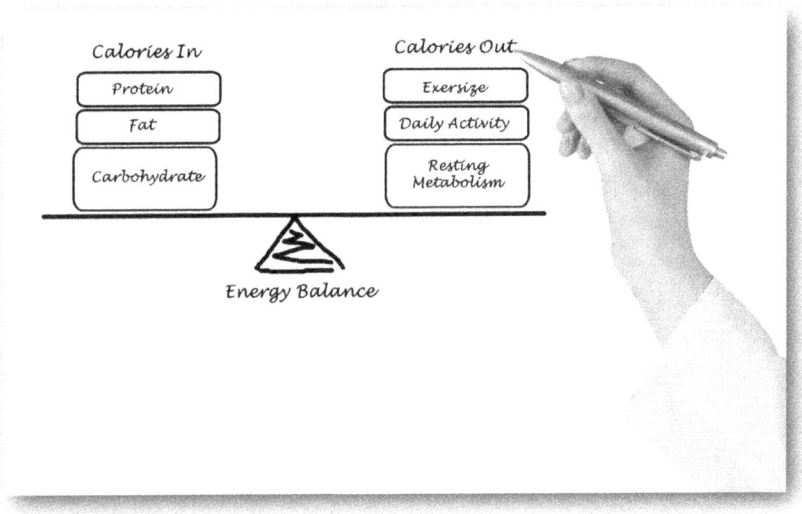

What Is Energy Balance?

It is important for us to understand the concept of energy balance. Energy balance refers to the relationship between *energy in* and *energy out*. Whatever you eat or drink is the energy in, and whatever your body burns through its core functions or physical activity is energy out.

Our bodies are always burning energy, even when we are asleep. As we increase physical activity, we consume more energy. If we eat and drink more in a day than our bodies need, we convert the excess energy into fat and store it. That is the essential reason for weight gain;

we gain those extra pounds because we have consumed more calories than our bodies need.

The reverse is also true when we are trying to lose weight. If we are consuming fewer calories than our bodies are using through physical exercise, we lose weight. That is because the body converts some of the stored fat back into energy to fuel our muscles and other organs.

In a single day, we may not notice a slight energy imbalance; however, if we do not maintain an energy balance over time, we can gain weight and damage our health. Since children are also growing, they use energy differently. They use some of the energy in to support the growth of vital body tissues. However, if too many calories are taken in through food and beverages, they can add weight quickly.

The US Department of Health and Human Services, in conjunction with the Department of Agriculture, has developed a valuable chart to show our estimated calorie requirements. The estimates are rounded to the nearest 200 calories and were determined using an equation from the Institute of Medicine.[11].

Table 3.

Estimated Calorie Requirements (in kilocalories) for Each Gender
and Age Group at Three Levels of Physical Activity.

Gender	Age (years)	Activity Level		
		Sedentary	Moderately Active	Active
Child	2-3	1,000	1,000 - 1,400	1,000 - 1,400
Female	4 - 8	1,200	1,400 - 1,600	1,400 - 1,800
Female	9-13	1,600	1,600 - 2,000	1,800 - 2,000
Female	14-18	1,800	2,000	2,400
Female	19-30	2,000	2,000 - 2,200	2,400
Female	31-50	1,800	2,000	2,200
Female	51+	1,600	1,800	2,000 - 2,200
Male	4-8	1,400	1,400 - 1,600	1,600 - 2,000
Male	9-13	1,800	1,800 - 2,200	2,000 - 2,600
Male	14-18	2,200	2,400 - 2,800	2,800 - 3,200
Male	19-30	2,400	2,600 - 2,800	3,000
Male	31-50	2,200	2,400 - 2,600	2,800 - 3,000
Male	51+	2,000	2,200 - 2,400	2,400 - 2,800

Source: HHS/USDA Dietary Guidelines for Americans: 2005

Consider this. If you eat an extra 150 calories per day above your daily calorie requirements, you will may gain more than fifteen pounds per year. If you don't want that to happen, you have choices to make. You can reduce the number of calories consumed, or you can increase the number burned.

Small dietary changes can account for that 150-calorie reduction. These can include drinking water instead of a twelve-ounce regular soda or eating six ounces of tuna canned in water instead of in oil. Now, that wouldn't be hard, would it?

Small changes in physical activity can burn up those 150 calories in a hurry. You could do it by walking a couple of miles, doing some yard work, going for a bike ride, or climbing the stairs instead of using the elevator. The easiest way to maintain that energy balance so that you lose weight instead of gaining it is to do both; lose weight by reducing calories in and increasing calories out.

Are All Calories Equal?

Let's compare the calories from fresh vegetables and a carbonated beverage or fruit juice. The fresh vegetables contain fiber. The fiber reduces the number of calories absorbed by the body. The calories from the fresh vegetables that do get absorbed will be absorbed slowly, and they will not spike your blood sugar or insulin. Because of the fiber in the fresh vegetables, your stomach will also send a signal to your brain telling you to stop eating because you are full. The fresh vegetables also contain macro- and micronutrients that optimize your metabolism, lower cholesterol, reduce inflammation, and boost detoxification.

The beverage does not include fiber, vitamins, minerals, or phytonutrients to help you process the calories you are consuming. These are empty calories devoid of any nutritional value. The carbonated beverages and fruit juices usually contain fructose. This goes right to your liver, where it starts manufacturing fat, which triggers more insulin resistance and causes chronically elevated blood insulin levels, driving your body to store belly fat. You also get a fatty liver, which generates more inflammation. Chronic inflammation causes more weight gain and obesity.[12]

What I am trying to illustrate here is that *all calories are not created equal.* The same number of calories from different types of food can have very different biological effects on the body. According to Dr. Mark Hyman, you can see calories are different; some may be addictive, others healing, some fattening, some metabolism boosting. Switching to a plant-based whole-food diet can eliminate any chance of consuming empty calories.

Notes

[1]   Harvard T. H. Chan School of Public Health. 2016. "Fiber." *The Nutrition Source.* https://www.hsph.harvard.edu/nutritionsource/carbohydrates/fiber/.

[2]   World Health Organization. 2010. "Nutrient Profiling: Report of a WHO/IASO Technical Meeting. October 4–6. http://www.who.int/entity/nutrition/publications/profiling/WHO_IASO_report2010.pdf?ua=1.

[3]   Hunter, J. G., and K. L. Cason. 2006. "Nutrient Density." *Clemson University.* November. http://www.clemson.edu/extension/hgic/food/nutrition/nutrition/dietary_guide/hgic4062.html.

[4]   "Nutrient Profiling." See note 2.

[5]   Academy of Nutrition and Dietetics. 2014. "Vitamin and Nutrient Information from the Academy."

[6]   Hunter and Cason. See note 3.

[7]   Ibid.

[8]   Centers for Disease Control and Prevention. 2016. "Low-Energy-Dense Foods and Weight Management: Cutting Calories While Controlling Hunger." Accessed May 20. http://www.cdc.gov/nccdphp/dnpa/nutrition/pdf/r2p_energy_density.pdf.

[9]   Fuhrman, Joel. "Dr. Fuhrman's Nutritarian Pyramid." *DrFuhrman.com.* Accessed September 20. https://www.drfuhrman.com/library/foodpyramid.aspx.

[10] Ibid.

[11] National Heart, Lung, and Blood Institute. 2013. "Balance Food and Activity." *National Institutes of Health.* Accessed June 28. http://www.nhlbi.nih.gov/health/educational/wecan/healthy-weight-basics/balance.htm.

[12] Hyman, Mark. 2014. *The Blood Sugar Solution 10-Day Detox Diet,* 39–43. New York, NY: Little, Brown and Company.

CHAPTER 2

Is Overeating Associated with Bad Health?

mpty Eating is one of the habits contributing to weight gain. Another equally important factor is overeating. Most people know overeating isn't good for them. Obviously, it causes weight gain, and many complications arise from those extra pounds. Many have also misunderstood the causes of overeating and the devastating ways it affects the body. Honestly, we are often incapable of spotting overeating in our own lives.

As mentioned in the previous chapter, different foods have different caloric values. The number of calories in a particular amount of food determines how much energy that food introduces into the body when we eat it. As seen in table 1 in the last chapter, we have limits to the number of calories we should consume each day. Adding exercise increases the number of calories we can eat without gaining weight.

Overeating is consuming more calories than we need to maintain our body's health and to fuel physical activity.[1] In the United States, we have developed bad eating habits that include overeating at every meal. In the next few pages, let's explore the nature of overeating and why some people can't seem to control it.

Overeating can lead to eating disorders with serious health implications. If you're unsure whether you may be affected by overeating, here are some questions to consider:

- Do you feel out of control when eating?
- Do you think about food all the time?
- Do you eat in secret?
- Do you eat until you feel sick?
- Do you eat to escape from worries, relieve stress, or comfort yourself?
- Do you feel disgusted or ashamed after eating?
- Do you feel powerless to stop eating, even though you want to?[8]

If you answered yes to more than two of these questions, it is very likely that you are susceptible to overeating, or you may already be there.

However, overeating can be the result of several disorders: compulsive overeating, binge eating, and excessive hunger. Food addiction could also be included in this list, although some scientists think food addiction is involved in all the other conditions. Although these disorders have different causes and produce different behaviors, the result is the same. All forms of overeating cause weight gain.

Compulsive overeating, binge eating, and excessive hunger are all linked. A person suffering from compulsive eating can also indulge in binge eating and extreme hunger. Let's examine these disorders that lead to overeating, as well as their underlying causes.

Compulsive overeating occurs when someone does not feel hunger or has no physical need for food but eats anyway. Many people practice this to a minor extent. You may occasionally eat a candy bar when you don't feel hungry or have dessert after a meal when you are already full. That is compulsive eating. You may take a trip to the refrigerator, not because you are hungry, but because you are bored. Has this ever happened to you?

A compulsive eater behaves this way all the time. He or she eats on impulse without any other reason. This behavior suggests those with this condition are also obsessed with food. When not eating, they often think about what to eat next. Haslam and James, who wrote about obesity in the Lancet, a medical journal in the United Kingdom, claim that

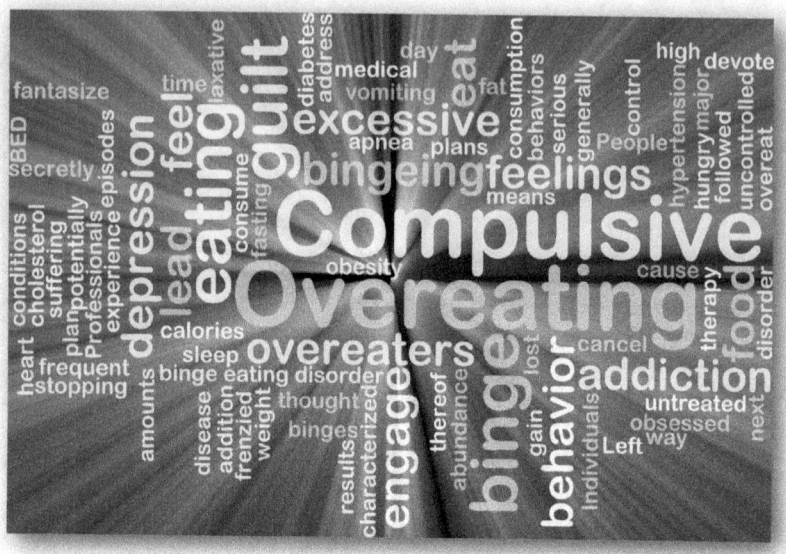

compulsive overeating is a serious matter that can easily lead to obesity and other complications, which can include kidney disease, arthritis, bone deterioration, and stroke in addition to high cholesterol, diabetes, heart disease, hypertension, sleep apnea, and major depression.[2]

Signs that a person is suffering from compulsive eating include rapid weight gain, frequently eating alone, eating large portions, or binge eating. Binge eating involves consuming several meals' worth of food in a single sitting. These episodes of lost self-control can cause emotional withdrawal and a feeling of guilt, followed by a period of inactivity and avoiding of social contact.[2] People who suffer from compulsive eating often feel shame and guilt over what they are doing. People closest to them may notice this behavior.

Compulsive eating can have several causes, mostly of an emotional nature. The Mayo Clinic staff claims that overeating is what they refer to as "emotional overeating."[3] Many of us have experienced emotional overeating when we were stressed and turned to food for comfort. Although this behavior is not very healthy, doctors don't consider it a disorder, just a coping mechanism. When comfort eating continues for an extended period, however, it may become a compulsive eating disorder. Compulsive eating may become so dangerous that it requires the attention of a psychologist with specialized training.

Binge eating is different from compulsive eating in that a person who engages in binge eating can have days of normal behavior, when his or her self-control is high enough, followed by episodes of extreme overeating, in which his or her restraint is entirely lost. People who have episodes of binge eating may eat up to 10,000 calories in a single meal. For most of us, that amount is as much as five days' worth of food in a healthy diet.

There can be several reasons for binge eating, some of them similar to what causes compulsive eating. Often, it is a response to stress or distress, such as emotional pain or anxiety. After several investigations into binge eating, Tuschl who wrote in an international research journal named Appetite that specializes in cultural, social, psychological, sensory and physiological influences on the selection and intake of foods and drinks, claims binge eating happens most often to people who try to limit their calories with a special restrictive diet, meaning they eat a lot less then they should.[4] When people radically reduce the amount of food they eat, as those on restrictive diets do, the body begins entering starvation mode. At this point, no significant physiological change, such as ketosis, is happening. Psychologically, however, starvation mode inflames appetite, making the person crave a lot more food.

When people lose self-control, they do not just overeat; they begin stuffing themselves with everything available. After the episode of binge eating is finished, people most often feel shame, guilt, and regret. Those emotional reactions can intensify the stress of compulsive eating, leading to even worse problems.

Excessive hunger is different from compulsive eating or binge eating in that the people suffering from excessive hunger genuinely feel hungry. Various influences, some of them physical health issues, can cause excessive hunger. Excessive hunger can result from a hormonal imbalance, an enlarged stomach, or a brain disorder.[5] Appetite determines how much we eat, but our brains and stomachs control appetite itself; when the stomach is full, it sends a signal to the brain within a short amount of time (a few minutes) saying you've eaten enough. That stops the appetite—at least in healthy, normal people.[6] Some health issues, such as diabetes, Kleine-Levin syndrome, and Prader-Willi syndrome, as well as certain hormonal imbalances, can disable this system.[7] Individuals who have a constant hunger that seems impossible to satisfy should consult their physicians for a physical examination.

Stress plays an important part in most, if not all, eating disorders. Emotional distress and pressure can make us seek comfort and emotional safety in food. Maintaining good physical health helps reduce all forms of stress, and decreased stress will make weight loss easier by reducing excessive eating patterns. To lose weight and keep a healthy body, consider the following ways to lower stress.

According to Dr. Neal Barnard of the Physicians Committee for Responsible Medicine, who published the article "How to Eat Right to Reduce Stress," eating high-fiber, carbohydrate-rich foods causes the brain to produce more serotonin, a hormone that relaxes us. Dr. Barnard also writes that eating antioxidant-rich fruits and vegetables can boost our immune system and weaken chronic stress.

Food Addiction—Addicted to Empty Calories

In addition to stress, other important factors influence weight gain. Empty calories and large portion sizes combine as two of the worst contributors to poor health.

Bearing that in mind, most empty calories come from highly processed foods that contain a lot of sugars and fats but have few, if any, nutrients. Eating these foods increases our weight. Now, let us consider why empty calories lead to overeating.

An increasing number of Americans are overweight or obese, seemingly incapable of losing weight. Some experts think the primary factor behind this trend is food with empty calories. Foods containing more fats, sugars, and salt seem to be more attractive to people than do healthier foods such as fruits, vegetables, and whole grains without added fats or sugars. Why is this so?

Our brains seem to be wired to crave unhealthy foods more than healthy foods.[7] When our brains evolved, our ancestors ate as much sugar and fat as they could, because it was rare and not easily obtainable.[8] Because life was so physically demanding, they needed all the energy they could get.

Thanks to modern technology, a greater variety of these foods is available to nearly everyone in the developed world. Most of us have succumbed to the temptation to indulge in these fattening foods on more than one occasion. Foods with added fat, salt, and sugar do taste better. Such foods are referred to as "super palatable," which means "super tasty."[9] In truth, nearly all snacks, sweets, and fast foods contain high levels of empty calories. At the same time, they are the most appealing foods on the menu. The theory makes sense if you think about it.

The foods we eat the most are the ones that produce the most weight gain. The very nature of these energy-dense foods causes people to overeat, at least in some cases. Everyone has that one unhealthy vice, the food we just can't stop eating. When we literally can't control our eating, we start to overeat. The combination of excess calories and empty calories guarantees an unhealthy body, weight gain, and in many cases obesity.[7]

Controlling overeating can be a tough task. For most people, losing weight depends directly on managing appetite, avoiding Empty Eating, and resisting overeating. In later chapters, we shall explore strategies to avoid gaining weight and Empty Eating in detail. Some easy tips on how to avoid overeating are as follows:

- **Manage your stress.** Since one of the main reasons for overeating is stress, try to find ways to cope with stress and emotional imbalances other than eating. Try exercise or meditation, or find a hobby that distracts you from thinking about food.

- **Try to eat more meals a day, and choose healthy snacks.** Everyone is different, so not everyone should eat the same number of meals per day. However, eating breakfast is paramount, because it jump-starts your metabolism in the morning, making for an excellent beginning. All the rest of your meals should contain as many different kinds of plant-based food as possible. As stated in the previous chapter, the healthiest foods are vegetables, whole grains, fruits, nuts, and seeds.
- **Remove the temptation by removing high-calorie, low-nutrient foods from the house.** If you have junk food, desserts, and unhealthy snacks in the house, the chances of you succumbing to temptation and eating them is high.
- **Stop dieting.** The deprivation and hunger of strict dieting can trigger food cravings and the urge to overeat. Instead of dieting, focus on eating healthy, whole foods. Find nutritious foods that you enjoy, and eat until you feel content and full. Eating low-calorie, high-nutrient foods and drinking a lot of water will help you avoid overeating. Many weight-loss specialists have suggested drinking one ounce of water for every pound of body weight. They dismiss the familiar "eight glasses a day" routine as being not enough for most people. Americans are notorious for being both dehydrated and overweight.
- **Increase activity.** Exercise aids weight loss, helps lift depression, improves overall health, and reduces stress. It can make you feel better on many levels.
- **Spot emotional hunger.** Learn to identify the difference between physical and emotional hunger. If you ate recently and don't have a rumbling stomach, you're probably not hungry. You may just be trying to manage boredom or stress with food.
- **Limit portion sizes.** Regardless of how many meals you eat a day, watch the portion sizes. Keep all portion sizes trending smaller than you would have previously.

Notes

[1] Haslam, D. W., and W. P. James. 2005. "Obesity." *The Lancet* 366 (9492): 1197–209. doi: 10.1016/S0140-6736(05)67483-1.

[2] Ibid.

[3] Mayo Clinic Staff. 2015. "Weight Loss: Gain Control of Emotional Eating." *Mayo Clinic.* October 3. Accessed September 20. http://www.mayoclinic.org/healthy-living/weight-loss/in-depth/weight-loss/art-20047342.

[4] Tuschl, Reinhard J., Reinhold G. Laessle, Petra Platte, and Karl-Martin Pirke. 1990. "Differences in Food-Choice Frequencies between Restrained and Unrestrained Eaters." *Appetite* 14 (1): 9–13. doi: 10.1016/0195-6663(90)90050-i.

[5] Berthoud, H. R., N. R. Lenard, and A. C. Shin. 2011. "Food Reward, Hyperphagia, and Obesity." *American Journal of Physiology: Regulatory, Integrative, and Comparative Physiology* 300 (6). doi: 10.1152/ajpregu.00028.2011.

[6] Fulton, S. 2010. "Appetite and Reward." *Frontiers in Neuroendocrinology* 31 (1): 85–103. doi: 10.1016/j.yfrne.2009.10.003.

[7] Berthoud et al. See note 5.

[8] Kessler, David. 2010. *The End of Overeating: Taking Control of the Insatiable American Appetite.* New York, NY: Rodale Books.

[9] Ibid.

CHAPTER 3

What Overeating Does to Our Bodies

O vereating seems to be more common than most people realize. Now that we have defined it, we can examine the devastating impact overeating has on our bodies. Overeating, especially when we're consuming empty calories, causes many health complications. Undeniably, the most common health risks caused by overeating are weight gain and obesity. Eating too much food causes people to take in too much energy, which the body then converts into fat stores.[1]

I realize this may seem obvious, but in a majority of cases, weight gain is a direct consequence of eating too much food. People who eat too much usually eat the wrong foods, too.

Being overweight or obese causes a variety of health problems.

As you can see in table 3, the National Center for Health Statistics shows an average of 62 percent increase in the obesity among men and an average of 67 percent increase in obesity among women in the years studied. Reducing Empty Eating will slow down and even reverse obesity resulting from overeating.

Between 1988 and 1994 and between 2007 and 2008, the prevalence of obesity among adults at all levels of education increased, according to the US Department of Health and Human Services, Centers for Disease Control and Prevention, and National Center for Health Statistics.

Table 3. Prevalence of obesity among adults aged twenty years and older, by education and sex

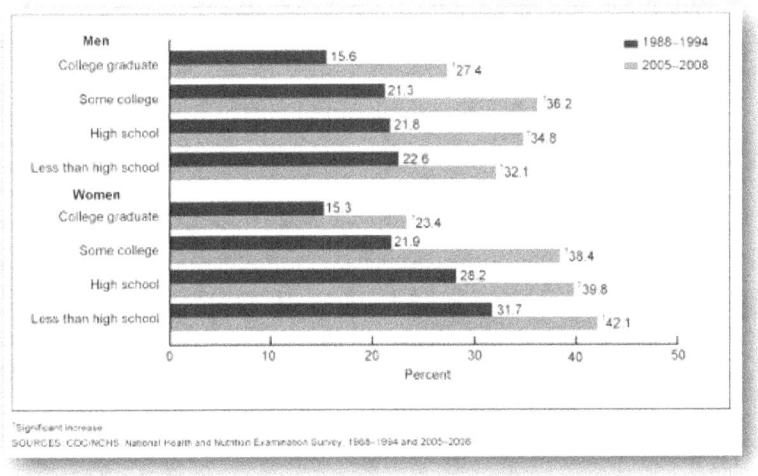

Whatever the reason for overeating and obesity, they cause many diseases and conditions, the most severe of which include type 2 diabetes, cardiovascular diseases, and certain types of cancer; collectively, doctors call these conditions metabolic syndrome.[2]

Metabolic syndrome refers to a combination of symptoms people have simultaneously, often as the consequence of obesity and overeating. The symptoms include the buildup of abdominal fat, high blood pressure, elevated levels of blood sugar, high levels of cholesterol, and high levels of triglycerides.[3] When at least three of these are present, doctors consider the patient to have metabolic syndrome. Metabolic syndrome increases the patient's risk of developing cardiovascular disease, particularly heart failure, and diabetes.

A number of factors can cause metabolic syndrome, but the condition is most often related to chronic overeating and obesity. The International Diabetes Federation Task Force on Epidemiology and Prevention; the National Heart, Lung, and Blood Institute; the American Heart Association; the World Heart Federation; the International Atherosclerosis Society; and the International Association for the Study of Obesity all agree on the guidelines for identifying metabolic syndrome and agree that metabolic syndrome is the number-one health risk for obese people.[4]

Several factors contribute to developing metabolic syndrome. Chronic overeating, a lack of physical activity, an unhealthy diet, stress, and some genetic factors all contribute to its development.[5]

Type 2 diabetes, or insulin-resistant diabetes, was known as *adult-onset diabetes* until recently, because it was unheard of for children to develop this condition. In the past few decades, this has changed, because so many children grow up overweight or obese. The rise of the disease in younger populations has resulted in the name change to *type 2 diabetes*.[6] The World Health Organization estimates that more than twenty million Americans, or 7 percent of the population, have type 2 diabetes. Unfortunately, about 6.2 million of those people do not even know they have it at its early stages.[7]

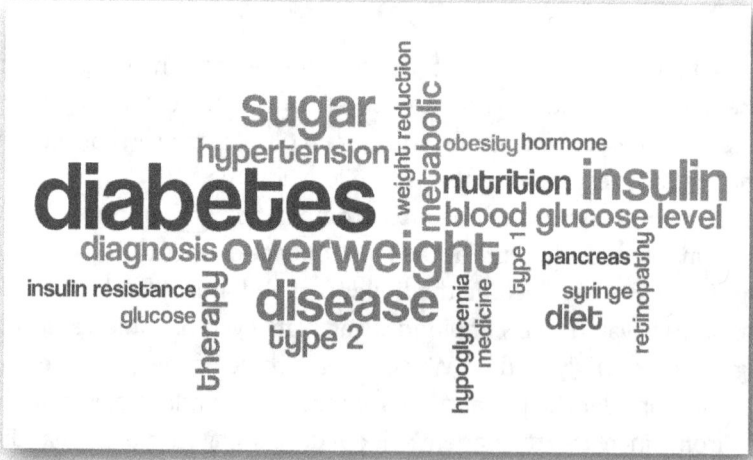

Diabetes interferes with the body's ability to use insulin, and insulin is necessary to keep blood sugar under control. When we eat too much, our bodies become flooded with insulin, which in turn causes our cells and organs to become more resistant to insulin.[8] This leads to more sugar in the blood but less sugar in the cells, and this rise in blood sugar means the cells of the body are not eating the sugar and in fact are starving, because they did not receive the signal from insulin to eat the sugar that is accessible in the blood. In their paper on obesity, Haslam and James cite diabetes as the cause of even more health problems, including kidney disease, eye problems or blindness, or nerve damage to the feet that can lead to amputation. Other complications include nerve disorders, skin problems, delayed gastric emptying, and an increased risk of heart attacks and cardiovascular problems.[9] Increased hunger, usually right after one has eaten, is one of the signs of diabetes and one of the main reasons people with diabetes overeat.

Coronary artery disease is one of the significant risks of overeating. Being overweight, having diabetes, having high cholesterol, and having high blood pressure are all risk factors for this disorder, which causes the narrowing of arteries that supply blood to the heart.[10] Coronary artery disease is the root cause of some heart problems, including angina, heart attacks, heart failure, and irregular heartbeat, as well as being a critical factor in strokes.[11] Diseases of the blood vessels can also lead to pulmonary embolism, which is a counterpart of strokes, with a blood clot traveling to the lungs and obstructing blood from reaching the lungs.[12] About fifteen million people have coronary artery disease, and it causes almost half a million deaths per year in the United States, making it one of the country's greatest killers.

Strokes are the third leading cause of death in the United States and, more often than not, are a consequence of obesity.[13] They occur when a blood clot blocks an artery or a blood vessel breaks in the neck or head, interrupting blood flow to part of the brain. When this happens, cells suffer from oxygen deprivation, causing brain cells to die and

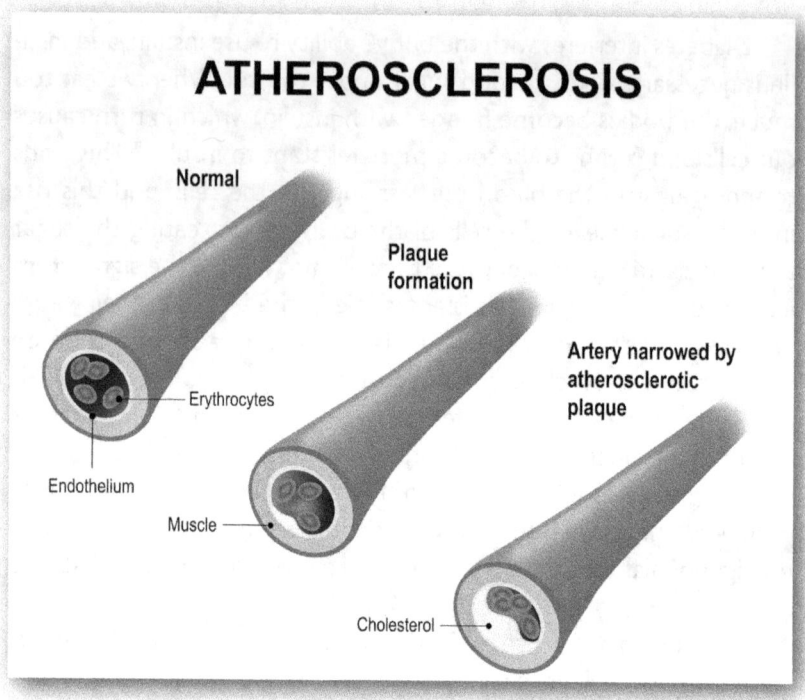

ATHEROSCLEROSIS

Normal

Plaque formation

Artery narrowed by atherosclerotic plaque

Erythrocytes

Endothelium

Muscle

Cholesterol

brain damage to begin right away. Depending on where in the brain the stroke occurs and how big the blood vessels are, it may affect memory, movement, or speech. A minor stroke may cause only weakness in the limbs; however, a major stroke can paralyze its victim, leaving him or her unable to speak or function. In some cases, a stroke can lead to death. High blood pressure, high cholesterol, diabetes, and excess weight are the most important risk factors for strokes. Many stroke sufferers can trace these associated health risks back to overeating.

Cancer is another of the diseases heavily correlated with obesity. Several studies of various types of cancer have linked obesity and overeating.[14] The National Cancer Institute reports that obesity and overeating may increase one's risk of esophageal cancer, as well as increasing the chances one may suffer from cancers of the breast (postmenopausal), endometrium (the lining of the uterus), colon and rectum, kidney, pancreas, thyroid, or gallbladder, among others. One

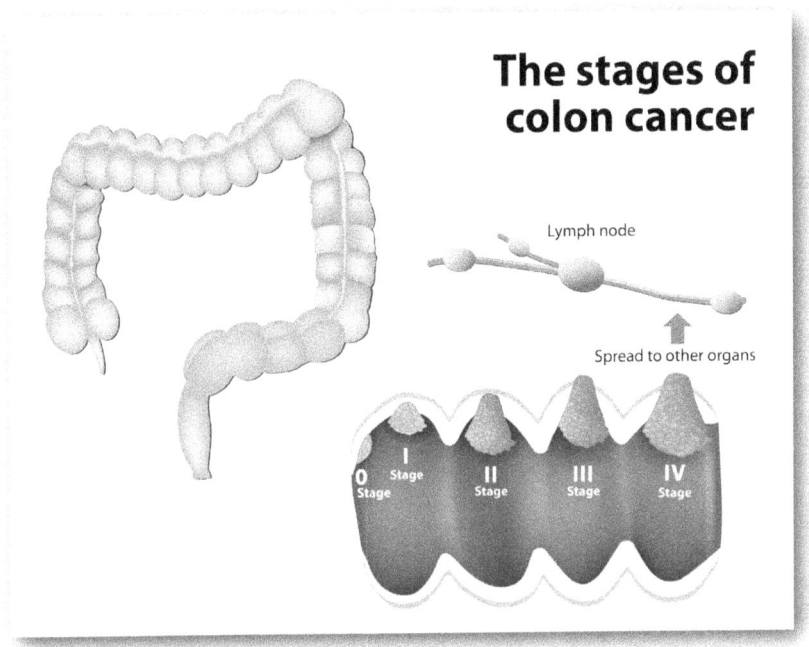

The stages of colon cancer

Lymph node

Spread to other organs

Stage 0   Stage I   Stage II   Stage III   Stage IV

study, conducted by the National Cancer Institute, estimated that in 2007 in the United States, about 34,000 new cases of cancer in men (4 percent) and 50,500 in women (7 percent) were due to obesity. The percentage of cases of cancer that were the consequence of obesity were different for various cancer types, but it was as high as 40 percent for some, particularly cancer of the uterus and of the esophageal lining.[15] This means that obese people have 40 percent exposure to some cancer types.

Overeating and obesity also cause some diseases of the digestive tract and its associated systems. Our bodies are not meant to contain, digest, and absorb so much food at one time; therefore, many systems related to food often stop functioning properly due to overeating.

Gastroesophageal reflux disease, or GERD, is a result of overeating. It occurs when patients sustain stomach-acid damage to the upper digestive tract and the esophagus.[16] This deterioration happens because the upper barrier that protects the esophagus from the stomach acid stops functioning properly. The barrier consists of a muscle ring (the lower esophageal sphincter), and the ring weakens when people overeat and a stomach full of food puts more pressure on it. Chronic overeating causes the esophageal sphincter to decline further and, at some point, to stop functioning properly. GERD causes many adverse effects, such as stomach and chest pain, bad breath, reflux, coughing, and occasional vomiting. Finally, after the esophagus sustains enough damage, GERD can lead to cancer.[17]

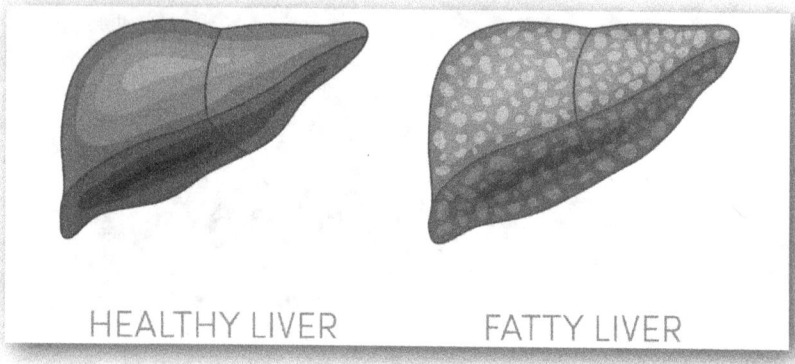

HEALTHY LIVER   FATTY LIVER

Fatty liver disease usually results from alcohol abuse; however, in some cases, overeating and its ensuing conditions may cause fatty liver. Abnormal fat deposits in the liver and clotting lead to weaker liver function, and the disease can lead to a form of jaundice and the buildup of toxins in the body. Fatty liver disease usually goes hand in hand with metabolic syndrome (a state that leads to obesity) and an insulin resistance.[4] Research shows consumption of excess amounts of carbonated beverages may result in fatty liver disease.[18]

Gallstones are another side effect of overeating and excess body weight. Gallstones form in the gallbladder, an accessory organ to digestion, from gall salts. The bile the gallbladder produces serves to aid digestion of fats in the small intestine. Once formed, gallstones cause pain, discomfort, digestion problems, and inflammation. In critical cases, gallstones can burst the gallbladder, releasing bile into the surrounding organs.[4] When gallstones are formed, the gallbladder should be monitored, and if the problem persists, the gallbladder may need to be removed surgically. People with no gallbladder have problems digesting fats, making diet choices afterward much more complicated.[19] Some risk factors leading to gallstones include the following:

- Being overweight or obese
- Eating a high-fat or high-cholesterol diet
- Rapid weight loss within a short period of time
- Having diabetes

Sleep apnea is another condition associated with obesity. The Mayo Clinic defines sleep apnea as a potentially dangerous sleep disorder causing breathing complications. You may have sleep apnea if you snore loudly, feel tired even after a full night's sleep, or gasp in the middle of the night. There are two types of sleep apnea, obstructive and central.

Obstructive sleep apnea is the more common form, which occurs when throat muscles relax. Researchers have related obstructive sleep apnea to obesity.

Central sleep apnea occurs when the brain doesn't send proper signals to the muscles that control breathing. The signs and symptoms of obstructive and central sleep apneas overlap, sometimes making the diagnosis of sleep apnea difficult.

The most common signs and symptoms of obstructive and central sleep apneas include these:

- Excessive sleep
- Loud snoring
- Pauses in breathing during sleep
- Waking and gasping
- Waking with a dry mouth or a sore throat
- A headache in the morning
- Difficulty staying asleep

People usually do not consider snoring a big problem, so they do not seek medical attention when it may be needed. Sleep apnea can lead to complications such as high blood pressure, fatigue, and problems with the liver.[20]

Obesity and overeating may also cause several psychological problems. As mentioned in the previous chapters, research has linked overeating to depression, mood changes, social isolation, and a general lack of psychological well-being.[21] People who are obese or who over-eat report more depression, lack of motivation, and social problems. This further contributes to the problems by strengthening the already negative effects of obesity and overeating. It becomes a vicious cycle. A person who suffers from depression is less likely to do something to change his or her life. This would further contribute to his or her obesity, resulting in further depression.[22]

After we list all the negative effects overeating can have on our health, it becomes apparent that we must do everything possible to escape these dreadful conditions.

Notes

[1] National Heart, Lung, and Blood Institute. 1998. "Clinical Guidelines on the Identification, Evaluation, and Treatment of Overweight and Obesity in Adults." NHLBI Obesity Education Initiative Expert Panel. Accessed September 20, 2016. http://www.nhlbi.nih.gov/guidelines/obesity/ob_gdlns.pdf.

[2] Ford, E. S., W. H. Giles, and W. H. Dietz. 2002. "Prevalence of Metabolic Syndrome among US Adults: Findings from the Third National Health and Nutrition Examination Survey." *Journal of the American Medical Association* 287.

[3] Ibid.

[4] Alberti, K. G., et al. 2009. "Harmonizing the Metabolic Syndrome: A Joint Interim Statement of the International Diabetes Federation Task Force on Epidemiology and Prevention; National Heart, Lung, and Blood Institute; American Heart Association; World Heart Federation; International Atherosclerosis Society; and International Association for the Study of Obesity." *Circulation* 120 (16).

[5] Ford et al. See note 2.

[6] Melmed, Shlomo, K. S. Polonsky, P. R. Larsen, and H. M. Kronenberg. 2011. *Williams Textbook of Endocrinology*, 12th ed., 1371–1435. Philadelphia: Elsevier/Saunders.

[7] Alberti et al. See note 4.

[8] Melmed et al. See note 6.

[9] Haslam, D. W., and W. P. James. 2005. "Obesity." *The Lancet* 366 (9492): 1197–209. doi: 10.1016/S0140-6736(05)67483-1.

[10] Ibid.

[11] Ibid.

[12] Ibid.

[13] Ibid.

[14] Dobbins, M., B. C. Choi, and K. Decorby. 2013. "The Association between Obesity and Cancer Risk: A Meta-Analysis of Observational Studies from 1985 to 2011." *ISRN Preventive*

Medicine. Accessed September 21, 2016. http://www.ncbi.nlm.nih. gov/pubmedhealth/PMH0069551/.

[15] http://www.cancer.gov/cancertopics/factsheet/Risk/obesity. https://www.cancer.gov/about-cancer/causes-prevention/risk/ obesity/obesity-fact-sheet#q3: Accessed September 21, 2016.

[16] Haslam. See note 9.

[17] Melmed et al. See note 6.

[18] Nseir, W., F. Nassar, and N. Assy. 2010. "Soft Drinks Consumption and Nonalcoholic Fatty Liver Disease." *World Journal of Gastroenterology* 16 (21).

[19] Melmed et al. See note 6.

[20] Mayo Clinic Staff. 2015. "Sleep Apnea." *Mayo Clinic.* August 25. Accessed September 21, 2016. http://www.mayoclinic.org/ diseases-conditions/sleep-apnea/basics/definition/con-20020286.

[21] Melmed et al. See note 6.

[22] Roberts, R. E. 2003. "Prospective Association between Obesity and Depression: Evidence from the Alameda County Study." *International Journal of Obesity* 27: 514–521. Accessed September 21, 2016. doi: 10.1038/sj.ijo.0802204.

CHAPTER 4

Is Intermittent Fasting the Solution?

There are many weight-loss and health-boosting diets out there: no fat, all fat, low carb, cabbage soup, six small meals, raw veggies no dressing, gluten free, etc. Restrictive diets (diets with fewer calories than standard nutrition) are the most common way for people to try to lose weight.

Most weight-loss diets restrict both the kinds and amounts of food you can eat. The actual plans vary from diets proposing that you avoid one food type to diets forcing another food type. Most diets, however, have shown themselves to be largely ineffective in the long term, as they often lead to a yo-yo effect, in which excess weight returns soon after the diet ends.

Most restrictive diets have a limited duration, during which dieters eat less than normal, so they lose weight; then they return to their regular diets. The act of eating less than usual causes the body to starve for nutrients for a while. During the period when the dieter consumes fewer calories, the body is in a constant state of stress, because it senses that food has become scarce.

When the dieter returns to a regular diet, the body tries to compensate for the period of limited food and lost weight by increasing its fat stores. This goes directly against the diet the dieter tried so hard to follow, and shortly after ending his or her diet, the dieter regains that lost weight, plus a few extra pounds. A 2007 study by Amigo and Fernandez explains that the yo-yo effect is common when people use restrictive diets to lose weight.[1] Such diets lead to a loss of muscle mass as well as fat, may result in malnutrition, and can cause many other adverse effects. A reduction in muscle mass means the body does not burn as many calories, so the body converts more of the excess calories to fat stores—ironically, you can lose weight while getting fatter.

One other negative factor to consider with restrictive diets is their effect on overeating and binge-eating disorders. Restrictive diets have a powerful effect on the emotional state of those practicing them. The limits imposed by such extreme diets cause effects such as depression or fatigue, making the diets almost impossible to sustain. Ultimately, the dieter reverts to his or her old eating habits, but now he or she feels depressed because of his or her failure to lose weight. Such an emotional state leads many people to eat more than they did before dieting, causing them to regain weight very quickly.[2]

Restrictive diets are only one of the ways to lose weight. Another way is gaining popularity fast, and it has potentially more beneficial effects. Intermittent fasting is a broad term, describing modes of diet that fall somewhere between fasting and regular eating. Fasting means not eating, or avoiding any calorie intake, for a specified period. The basis of intermittent fasting is having alternating periods of normal nutrition and fasting. Intermittent fasting methods vary in the length of their fasting and feeding periods. The basics of how fasting influences the body are the same, regardless of which strategy is used.

It seems that fasting can provide multiple health benefits desired by most people, including improved cardiovascular health, reduced cancer risk, insulin regulation, gene repair, and longevity.

Dr. Michael Mosley, in his feature documentary *Eat, Fast, and Live Longer*, claims we are eating too frequently, and that is causing a drop in general health, contributing to many diseases and disorders. When in constant "feast mode," your body forgoes much of its natural "repair and rejuvenation programming."

Diets based on severe calorie restriction promote both weight loss and longevity in animal models, but this kind of starvation diet is not a very appealing strategy for most people and also has the many adverse effects mentioned above.[3]

However, modern research shows that you can get most, if not all, the same benefits of severe calorie restriction with fewer detrimental consequences and less effort through intermittent fasting. Intermittent fasting is an eating schedule in which you feast during a particular time and reduce or stop eating during another period.

This kind of eating comes from the principle that our ancestors' diet looked very different from ours. Food was scarce back then, and only a few people ate rich food every day. Most people ate only occasionally, so they ate large portions when the opportunity arose.

Intermittent fasting finds its roots in the idea that eating a standard diet with the proper number of calories, with occasional periods of not eating, is more like that diet our ancestors had long ago. Supporters of intermittent fasting believe this is healthier and more natural for us. Some research shows that alternating periods of feasting and famine causes biochemical benefits in our bodies.[4] According to this theory, your body sees the effect not only of *what* you eat and *how* you eat it, but also of *when* you eat.

Intermittent fasting provides many health benefits, mostly related to metabolism, cardiovascular health, and nutrition-related health. One of the primary benefits of intermittent fasting is its effect on insulin and leptin metabolism.

Leptin is a "satiety hormone," produced by adipose (fat) cells to regulate energy balance by inhibiting hunger. In other words, it tells your brain when you have had enough food, so your appetite decreases. Intermittent fasting can regulate how leptin works; then the leptin hormone regulates appetite and reduces your craving for food.

Intermittent fasting also regulates insulin, leading to more efficient metabolism. This improves general health on several levels. It stimulates the body's cells to get the energy they need and leads to less fat buildup. Most importantly, regulating insulin levels helps prevent and treat diabetes and metabolic syndrome.[5]

Sugar (glucose) is the primary source of energy for your body, and the insulin hormone regulates how it is used. When too much glucose is present at all times because of overeating or a high-calorie diet, it can disturb the insulin balance in the body, leading to insulin resistance. Insulin resistance is one of the primary drivers of many diseases, from heart disease to cancer and, most of all, diabetes.[6]

Intermittent fasting helps reset your body to use fat as its primary fuel, and mounting evidence confirms that when your body becomes adapted to burning fats instead of sugar as its primary fuel, you dramatically reduce your risk of chronic disease. It also helps reduce the levels of blood sugar, reducing risks of insulin resistance.

Research has shown that fasting can raise human growth hormone (HGH) levels by as much as 1,300 percent in women and 2,000 percent in men. The human growth hormone plays an important part in health, fitness, and slowing the aging process. Researchers have tied HGH to burning fat stores and stimulating muscle growth as well; these functions help us lose fat and build muscle mass to achieve a lean look.[7] Fasting also potentially stimulates the immune system and contributes to a reduction in free radical buildup. Free radicals are active substances in the body created as waste from normal metabolic processes. Researchers have found to be some of the primary causes of cancer and other diseases.[8]

Numerous studies show that fasting has a beneficial impact on longevity in animals. Some experiments show that animals subjected to periodic fasting have much better general health and live about 30 percent longer.[9] This is probably due to the ability of intermittent fasting to regulate insulin metabolism and reduce free radicals, as well as its benefits to the cardiovascular system.

Considering all the effects intermittent fasting has on the body, it seems to be an effective way to lose weight, regulate our appetites, and gain better overall health.

Lastly, scientists have confirmed that fasting is beneficial for the prevention of dementia and other age-related neurodegenerative diseases. This probably comes from mechanisms such as support for the creation of ketones used by the brain as fuel rather than glucose. The nervous system also benefits from fasting's reduction of the production of free radicals in the body.[10]

In addition to preventing free radicals, intermittent fasting also boosts production of a protein called brain-derived neurotropic factor, which helps the brain produce new brain cells. It also protects brain cells from changes associated with Alzheimer's and Parkinson's diseases. Research by Dr. Mark Mattson, a senior investigator for the National Institute on Aging, suggests that alternate-day fasting (restricting your meal on fasting days to about 600 calories) can boost production of the factor by anywhere from 50 to 400 percent, depending on the brain region.[11]

Not everyone may benefit from all forms of intermittent fasting. If you are taking medication, you may want to check with your healthcare provider before adjusting your diet. However, several modern styles of intermittent fasting exist, and each may be suited for different people.

The first step in getting started is selecting the "mode" that works best for you. Each method has its own guidelines for how to fast and what to eat during the feeding phase. Below, we describe some of the most popular modes of intermittent fasting:

- **The UpDayDownDay™ Diet** or **The Alternate-Day Diet** or **Alternate-Day Fasting:** James Johnson, MD, developed this intermittent fasting method. Dr. Johnson recommends this method for disciplined people who are trying to lose weight and have a specific weight goal in mind. The basics of this diet are easy to follow: eat very little one day, and eat normally the next. On fasting days, you should eat less; your calorie intake should be around one-fifth of your typical diet. It is common for women to eat around 2,000 calories and for men to eat around 2,500 calories on regular days; therefore, on a fasting day, you should eat between 400 and 500 calories. Several tools on the Internet help people track how many calories they should eat in a day. One recommended application for this is the USDA supertracker tool (https://www.supertracker. usda.gov/default.aspx). On fasting days, Johnson recommends using meal-replacement shakes fortified with essential nutrients. You can sip these throughout the day, rather than splitting your food intake into small meals, which may help you feel less hungry during the day.[12]

- **The "Eat Stop Eat" method:** Brad Pilon developed the "Eat Stop Eat" method, which he suggests for healthy eaters looking for an extra boost. It consists of fasting for twenty-four hours once or twice per week. During the twenty-four-hour fast, which Pilon refers to as the "twenty-four-hour break from eating," dieters don't eat any food, but you can drink calorie-free beverages such as coffee, diet soda, and unsweetened, nonalcoholic beverages. After the fast is over, you go back to eating normally. You can end the fast with a large meal or a snack, depending on your preference.

  Eating this way will reduce overall calories consumed without limiting what you are able to eat—just how often you eat. It is important to note that incorporating regular workouts, particularly resistance training, is very beneficial for people trying to lose weight and gain a lean body.[13]

- **The "Leangains" method:** Martin Berkhan started the "Leangains" method, which is useful primarily for dedicated gym goers who want to lose body fat and build muscle. In this approach, Berkhan recommends fasting for fourteen hours each day for women and sixteen hours for men; the feeding period is the remaining six to eight hours. During the fasting period, you can consume no calories, though the method allows black coffee, calorie-free sweeteners, diet soda, and sugar-free gum. Most people find it easiest to fast through the night, while they sleep, and into the morning, breaking the fast roughly six hours after waking up; this reduces the period in which you feel hungry. Maintaining a consistent feeding window is important in this system to make sure that your hormones adapt and to make it easier to fast. What and when you eat during the feeding window also depends on when and how you work out. On the exercise days, carbohydrates are more important than fat. On the resting days, fat intake should be higher and carbohydrate consumption lower. You should eat high-protein foods every day, although the specific amounts depend on your gender, your age, and the specific goal you have in mind (losing weight or gaining muscle mass). Regardless of your particular program, whole, unprocessed foods should make up the majority of your calorie intake.[14]

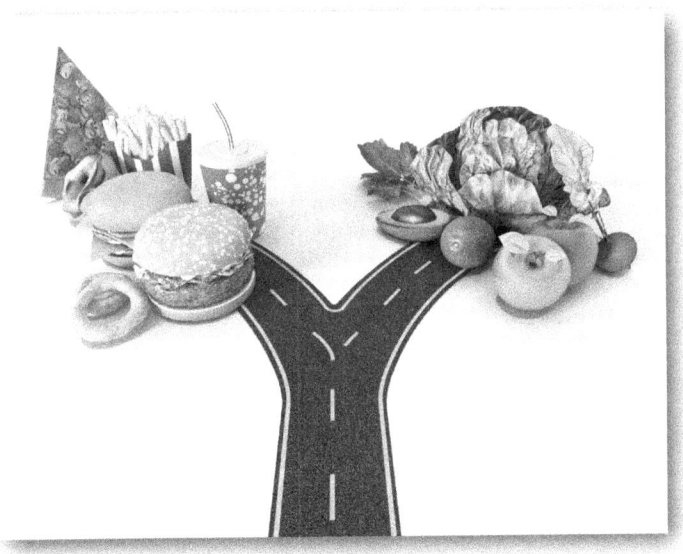

Considering the benefits provided by intermittent fasting when compared to other weight-loss and dieting plans, it seems that intermittent fasting may be good not only for weight loss and for regulating appetite and metabolism but also for general and overall health. It can be a very useful method for beating overeating and weight gain, and it is arguably easier to practice than other calorie-restriction diets.

Notes

[1] Amigo, I., and C. Fernandez. 2007. "Effects of Diets and Their Role in Weight Control." *Psychology, Health, & Medicine* 12.

[2] Ibid.

[3] Mosley, Michael, and Mimi Spencer. 2015. *The FastDiet: Lose Weight, Stay Healthy, and Live Longer with the Simple Secret of Intermittent Fasting.* New York, NY: Atria Books.

[4] Mattson, M. P. 2014. "Fasting: Molecular Mechanisms and Clinical Applications." *National Center for Biotechnology Information* 19. February 4. Accessed September 21, 2016. http://www.ncbi.nlm.nih.gov/pmc/articles/PMC3946160/.

[5] Antoni, Rona, et al. 2014. "The Effects of Intermittent Energy Restriction on Indices of Cardiometabolic Health." Accessed September 21, 2016. http://ibimapublishing.com/articles/ENDO/2014/459119/459119.pdf.

[6] Mayfield, Jennifer. 1998. "Diagnosis and Classification of Diabetes Mellitus: New Criteria." *American Academy of Family Physicians.* October 15. Accessed September 21, 2016. http://www.aafp.org/afp/1998/1015/p1355.html.

[7] "Study Finds Routine Periodic Fasting Is Good for Your Health, and Your Heart." 2011. *EurekAlert! Science News.* American Association for the Advancement of Science. Intermountain Medical Center Heart Institute. Accessed September 21, 2016. http://www.eurekalert.org/pub_releases/2011-04/imc-sfr033111.php.

[8] An overview of the role of free radicals in biology and of the use of electron-spin resonance in their detection may be found here: Rhodes, Christopher J., ed. 2000. *Toxicology of the Human Environment: The Critical Role of Free Radicals.* London: Taylor & Francis Limited.

[9] Carlson, A. J., and F. Hoelzel. 1946. "Apparent Prolongation of the Life Span of Rats by Intermittent Fasting." *The Journal of Nutrition* 31. Accessed September 21, 2016. http://openwritings.net/sites/default/files/excerpt/files/J.%20Nutr.-1946-Carlson-363-75.pdf.

[10]   Young, Emma. 2012. "Deprive Yourself: The Real Benefits of Fasting."
       New Scientist. November 14. Accessed September 21, 2016. https://
       www.newscientist.com/article/mg21628912.400-deprive-yourself-
       the-real-benefits-of-fasting?full=true.

[11]   Ibid.

[12]   Johnson, James B., and Donald R. Laub. 2008. "About the Book:
       The Story of *The Alternate-Day Diet.*" Accessed September 21,
       2016.   http://www.johnsonupdaydowndaydiet.com/html/book.
       html#alternate-day-diet.

[13]   Steer, Adam, and Brad Pilon. 2016. "In Just One Day This Simple
       Strategy Frees You from Complicated Diet Rules." *Eat – STOP –
       Eat.* Accessed September 21, 2016.
       http://www.eatstopeat.com/.

[14]   Berkhan, Martin. 2016. "Intermittent Fasting Diet for Fat Loss,
       Muscle Gain and Health." *Leangains.* Accessed May 21, 2016.
       http://www.leangains.com/.

CHAPTER 5
Making It Work for Me

What Do I Do Now?

Getting started may be the hardest part of changing our dietary choices. When I started, I had a drive to do something different because of my health. Since then, I have learned that not only am I benefiting myself, but when I look at the big picture, it is no longer possible for me to engage in Empty Eating. Eating a plant-based diet helps our environment, the economy, and humanity. Following a plant-based diet is an attainable solution for my health and for the health crises looming over this country.

I knew I needed to do something different, because I wasn't happy with myself. When I smoked cigarettes, I wanted to stop because it was taking a toll on my life. To my surprise, I was able to quit smoking completely. Yes, it was difficult, but today I feel much better. Right now, if you are reading this book, you also have a new challenge and need to get started. The good news is that what you want is attainable. As with all challenges, when you reach your goal, you'll be happier and healthier, and you'll be motivated to maintain the many benefits of living a healthy lifestyle. When you get started, you'll feel better. Don't wait any longer. Let's do this!

Transitioning to a Better Future

Here are my top five tips for making a smooth transition to the plant-based diet and eliminating Empty Eating:

- **Take it one meal at a time.** Don't worry about dinner parties, holidays, or the potluck next week. Let's focus on what you are going to eat today. Please don't overcomplicate things, and above all, don't worry; you'll be OK. In the next chapter, I will share meals you can make in fifteen minutes, tops. As you will see, a good-tasting, healthy meal can be as simple as bean, rice, greens, and salsa. You can also make a meal from hummus, a tortilla with lettuce and tomatoes, or refried beans with corn, rice, and a variety of vegetables. I'm getting hungry just thinking about it!

- **Eat your carbohydrates.** As Dr. John McDougall says, "since the beginning of time, different human civilizations have survived for thousands of years eating starches such as corn, rice, potatoes, and barley." The benefits of eating starches and all other carbohydrates, including fiber, are low-calorie, high-nutrient benefits. Grains, beans, nuts, and seeds are all rich in complex carbohydrates and fiber, and they form the base of most healthy diets. Fruits and vegetables are also carbohydrates, and eating them is an excellent way to optimize your health.

- **Eat freely.** The biggest advantage of eating a plant-based diet is that you can eat all you want. Fruits and vegetables have a lot of bulk, but your stomach only has a volume of about one liter; however, the stomach has the ability to expand, so it can hold as much as two to three times its size of food.[1] If you were to revert to eating high-calorie, low-nutrient foods, you could consume thousands of calories but still not fill your stomach. Picture that. You have consumed thousands of calories, but you are still hungry. For example, a pound of beef top-sirloin steak, trimmed to one-eighth inch of fat has 912 calories. The calorie breakdown is 57 percent fat, 0 percent carbs, and 43 percent protein.[2] Compare that to a pound of fresh kale, which has only 227 calories. The calorie breakdown is 12 percent fat, 71 percent carbs, and 17 percent protein.[3] At some point in our lives, most of us have eaten a steak with plenty of room left over in our stomachs to eat more food. Eating a plant-based diet means you can eat as much as you like without consuming excess calories.

- **Train your taste buds.** We can distinguish five primary taste sensations: salty, sour, sweet, bitter, and umami (a pleasant savory taste found in foods such as meat, cheese, and mushrooms). You may find it difficult to believe, but you can train your taste buds to accept new and different foods, even foods you do not like right now. Accomplishing this takes about six to eight weeks. Most of us probably prefer to eat a lot of sugary, fatty, and salty foods. When we do, we increase our chances of becoming addicted to these foods and having them dull our taste buds over time. In fact, the more you eat, the more you want. According to David Katz, MD, "The less of a food you eat, the less of it you need to maintain the same desire."[4] While eating healthy, we have several ways to train our taste buds to enjoy eating more plant-based food:
  - Mask the flavor of foods by adding small portions of the food you don't like to foods you do like. "Over time your brain forms a positive association with both tastes," says Alan Hirsch, MD.[5]
  - Try eliminating one food you know is terrible for you, and try adding something you know would be good for you.
  - Start introducing healthier, unprocessed foods you don't normally have, prepared in a variety of different ways.
- **Be adventurous.** As often as possible, eat fruits and vegetables you do not ordinarily eat. Try something new. For example, I

recently ate some jackfruit and discovered that the flavor of Juicy Fruit gum comes from jackfruit. There have been times when I was walking through the produce section of the supermarket and saw a fruit or vegetable that I had never seen before. If this happens to you, go outside your comfort zone and try it.

Simple Strategies that Lead to Change

1. Make a commitment.
2. Don't give up. (Remember, science proves it works.)
3. Make whole foods the foundation of your diet.
4. Don't worry about counting calories. (Healthy food has bulk and is full of nutrients.)
5. Eat a rainbow of colors. (Different colored fruits and vegetables are full of antioxidants.)
6. Hang out with like-minded people. (It's easier to change.)
7. Eat ten or more fresh fruits or vegetables daily. (All fresh fruits and vegetables provide a variety of nutrients.)
8. Drink plenty of water. I drink half my weight in ounces.
9. Cook at home. When dining out, it's hard to control what ingredients are being used in your food. Very few restaurants prepare food without adding salt, sugars, unhealthy fats, and damaging chemicals.
10. Avoid all animal products such as meat, fish, eggs, and cheese. They are high in calories and low in nutrients (i.e., Empty Eating).
11. Eliminate all oil. Most oil in liquid or solid form contains approximately 120 empty calories per tablespoon.
12. Eat fruit, starch, seeds, grains, vegetables, nuts, and legumes.
13. Use herbs and spices daily. All herbs and spices are full of antioxidants. Herbs and spices intensify natural flavors without adding calories.

14. Eliminate all processed foods. They are high in calories and low in nutrients.
15. Try new plant-based foods. All contain different amounts of nutrients.
16. Remove all junk food from your diet. (They have few nutrients and a lot of calories.)
17. Start reading labels. Labels tell you what you are eating.
18. Cook a new recipe each week. Variety keeps it interesting. Many overweight people have very little variety in the foods they eat. You will enjoy your new eating lifestyle more if it has more variety than your old one did.
19. Eat more meatless ethnic foods. Many cultures use different natural herbs and spices, and many have delicious vegetable meals.
20. Carry your food with you to ensure you are eating the foods you want. That way, you do not get trapped without an excuse. It allows you to say no to the McDonald's sign.

Some Pointers for Reading Labels

Modern technology has given us access to a wide range of foods year-round. Some of this is due to chemical preservatives, highly refined carbohydrates, and processed fats. To make the healthy changes recommended by this book, you will need to understand what you are putting in your mouth. To help you do that, I'm including a few tips on how to read labels.

When comparing calories and nutrients in two packaged foods, make sure the serving size is the same. Otherwise, you may have a distorted idea of how many calories you are consuming.

If the label contains words that are more than fifteen letters long and sound like they come from bottles in a laboratory, those aren't food. They are chemical preservatives, food coloring, artificial sweeteners, or stabilizing substances. Don't even pretend you are eating real food.

If the label contains words with the suffix -ose, those are forms of sugar. Some food packages are dishonest enough to say that the product is sugar-free, but a quick reading of the label shows that the product includes glucose, sucrose, high-fructose corn syrup, sucralose, etc. Sugar-free does not mean calorie-free. Reduced sugar does not mean that the number of calories is actually lower.[6]

Understand the differences among fats. *Saturated fat* is a solid at room temperature. You can find it most frequently in animal-based foods, such as meat, cheese, and milk. It is also present in tropical oils such as coconut oil, palm oil, and cocoa butter. Saturated fat can raise your blood cholesterol. *Trans fat* or *hydrogenated fat* has been highly processed. You'll find this in processed foods, bakery goods, and some salad dressings. I'll be blunt; this stuff is dangerous. *Monounsaturated fat* comes from avocados, nuts, and some vegetable oils, such as canola oil and olive oil. It helps lower bad cholesterol (LDL) and actually raises the good cholesterol (HDL). *Polyunsaturated fat* comes mainly from vegetable oils. It has two forms: omega-3 and omega-6 fatty acids. Omega-3 fatty acids come from soybean oil, canola oil, walnuts, and flaxseed, as well as cold-water fish and shellfish. Omega-6 fatty acids are mostly in liquid vegetable oils such as soybean oil, corn oil, and safflower oil.[7]

Nutrition Facts

Serving Size 100 g

Amount Per Serving

Calories 250   Calories from fat 10

% Daily Value*

Total Fat 4%	4%
Saturated Fat 1.5%	4%
Trans Fat	
Cholesterol 50mg	28%
Sodium 150mg	15%
Total Carbohydrate 10g	3%
Dietary Fiber 5g	
Sugars 3g	
Protein 16%	

Vitamin A 1%	•	**Vitamin C** 3%	
Calcium 2%	•	**Iron** 2%	

*Percent Daily Values are based on a 2,000 calorie diet. Your daily values may be higher or lower depending on your calorie needs.

According to Jeff Novick, MS, RDN, LDN, who released a DVD titled *Should I Eat That?* on how to read labels, you can read a label in three steps:

1. If calories from fat (CFF) are less than 20 percent, you can eat it. (Divide CFF from total number of calories.)

2. If the amount of sodium is equal to or less than the total number of calories, you can eat it.
3. Always check the ingredients.
   a. Avoid all saturated fats (butter, lard, chicken fat, cheese).
   b. Avoid partially hydrogenated vegetable oil.
   c. Avoid any added sugars listed among the first three ingredients.

What Do I Do When My Stomach Is Empty?

When your stomach is empty, you will have a feeling of discomfort or weakness caused by a lack of food, coupled with the desire to eat. That is the definition of hunger. Sometimes, however, when we feel the discomfort of hunger, it may not be true hunger. In his book, *Eat to Live*, Dr. Joel Fuhrman coined the terms *toxic hunger* and *true hunger*. Dr. Fuhrman explains toxic hunger and true hunger:

> Eating low-nutrient foods leads to toxic hunger and the desire to overconsume calories. The body becomes toxic when we continuously eat unhealthy food. When you stop eating toxic food, the body craves them. Symptoms of toxic hunger are headaches, fatigue, nausea, weakness, mental confusion and irritability, abdominal and esophageal spasm, and fluttering and cramping in the stomach. When you consume natural food, you will not have any discomfort on an empty stomach. After several weeks of eating healthy food and accumulating macro- and micronutrients, you will no longer experience the symptoms of toxic hunger and start to experience the symptoms of true hunger. True hunger is felt in the throat, neck and mouth, and its symptoms are enhanced taste sensation, increased salivation, and gnawing throat sensation.[8]

Notes

1   "Stomach." 2016. *Columbia Encyclopedia*. New York, NY: Columbia University Press. Retrieved June 16, 2016. http://www.encyclopedia.com/doc/1E1-stomach.html/.

2   "Calories in 1 Lb. of Beef Top Sirloin and Nutrition Facts." 2016. *FatSecret*. Accessed June 16, 2016. http://www.fatsecret.com/calories-nutrition/usda/beef-top-sirloin-(trimmed-to-1-8-fat)?portionid=36486&portionamount=1.000/.

3   "Calories in 1 Lb. of Kale and Nutrition Facts." 2016. *FatSecret*. Accessed June 10, 2016. http://www.fatsecret.com/calories-nutrition/usda/kale?portionid=48790&portionamount=1.000/.

4   Pagan, Camille Noe. 2014. "6 Tricks for Training Your Taste Buds to Crave Healthy Foods." *Women's Health*, November 26. Accessed June 10, 2016. http://www.womenshealthmag.com/weight-loss/how-to-retrain-your-taste-buds/.

5   Ibid.

6   Webb, Gary. 2014. *Lasting Weight Loss: What Have You Got to Lose?* CreateSpace Independent Publishing Platform.

7   Healthwise Staff. 2013. "Types of fats." *eMedicineHealth*. Accessed July 1, 2016. http://www.emedicinehealth.com/types_of_fats-health/article_em.htm.

8   Fuhrman, Joel. 2011. *Eat to Live*. New York, NY: Little, Brown and Company.

CHAPTER 6

Healthy Slim-Down Meals

Time-Saving Tips for Meal Preparation

The following is a list of convenient foods that will take fifteen minutes or fewer to cook. Enjoy!

Brown Rice + Black Beans + Kale + Salsa
Brown Rice + Black-eyed Peas + Corn + Salsa
Brown Rice + Tempeh + Frozen Mixed Vegetables + Bragg
Liquid Aminos
Pasta + Lentils + Broccoli + Marinara Sauce
Potato + Black Beans + Kale + Salsa
Quinoa + White Beans + Baby Spinach + Dried Apricots +
Balsamic Dressing
Quinoa + Black Beans + Bell Peppers + Italian Dressing
Quinoa + Tempeh + Diced Fresh Mango + Pico de Gallo
Sweet Potato + Black Beans + Corn + Tortilla + Spinach
+ Tomato + Hummus

Note: Any types of beans, fresh greens, fruits, peas, or potatoes are just as delicious to substitute.

My Favorite Meal

Yukon Potatoes (cubed) + Black Beans + Pico de Gallo + Broccoli + FiberMega (FiberMega is a blend of chia, flax, pumpkin, and sesame seeds that can be purchased online at *www.fibermega.com*.) I personally use FiberMega on my food at every meal.

Recipe and cooking method

tt = to taste

1 qt.	boiling water
1 ea.	broccoli crown, small
2 ea.	Yukon potatoes, small, diced in cubes
½ pkg.	mirepoix, frozen 12-oz. bag
1 can	black beans
tt	garlic
tt	pepper
tt	salsa (I purchase mine from the neighborhood Mexican grocery store, because they make it fresh every day.)

1. Place potatoes in boiling water.
2. Bring mirepoix to a boil in ¼ cup of water.
3. Add beans to the mirepoix and stir.
4. Season beans to taste.
5. When the potatoes have cooked for 3–4 minutes, add the broccoli to the water and continue to boil. (The broccoli and potatoes are cooking together; keep in mind the potatoes take longer to cook than the broccoli does.)
6. Check to see if the potatoes are done.
7. When the potatoes are done, remove from heat, drain, and plate the broccoli and potatoes.
8. Add beans to the plate.

9. Sprinkle beans with FiberMega.
10. Add fresh salsa to the beans and potatoes.
11. Serve.

If you can multitask, you can complete all these steps simultaneously, and you'll have your meal ready in fifteen minutes or fewer. The advantage is a low-calorie, high-nutrient, very filling, and tasty meal.

Fifteen-Minute Dishes

The challenge many of us have in our busy daily routines is taking the time to cook a healthy meal. Not all meals can be prepared from scratch in fewer than twenty minutes, but many can. To make a plant-based meal in a few minutes, here are some essential ingredients you should keep in your house at all times:

1. Canned tomatoes (crushed, diced, pureed, or whole), 28-oz. can
2. Canned beans, 14-oz. can
3. Frozen fruit or vegetables (mixed fruits and vegetables are OK)
4. Starchy vegetables (brown rice, corn, potatoes, sweet potatoes, etc.)
5. Herbs, spices, and seasonings

If you decide to purchase foods packaged for convenience, choose packages that are stored in sterile containers. Canned tomatoes are healthy for you as long as the tomatoes have minimal processing, such as those sold crushed, diced, pureed, or whole. It is always better to purchase no-salt or reduced-salt canned foods. You can always add salt at the table. Some starches, such as barley and dried beans, may take more than fifteen minutes to prepare. Canned beans are just as healthy as dried beans, although you may want to rinse the canned beans to remove the added salt in the juice. Companies blanch frozen vegetables before freezing, which speeds the cooking. If you eat pasta, use whole-wheat pasta. Finally, it is always better to grow your own herbs and spices, but if you do decide to purchase them, check the labels to make sure there is no salt added, especially to the herb and spice blends.

Prepackaged foods are not all healthy for you. The only canned foods I favor eating are beans and tomatoes. Most other canned foods have added salt and sugar, not to mention the preservatives added to increase the shelf life of the product. The biggest advantages when using these foods are that you can make all your meals quickly and inexpensively in fifteen to twenty minutes with limited preparation, and cleanup is quick and easy.

Other advantages of using the foods listed above are that you can make all of them into healthy meals, and all are low in calories but high in nutrients. You don't have to worry about Empty Eating, and you can eat as much as you like.

Curry Vegetables

1 pkg.	mirepoix, 12 oz. frozen
8 oz.	water
1 can	diced tomatoes, 14 oz.
1 can	garbanzo beans, 14 oz.
1 lb.	frozen cauliflower
½ lb.	frozen peas
4 oz.	frozen kale or collard greens
2 ea.	potatoes, ½-inch cubed
2 tsp.	garam masala
tt	curry powder
tt	salt and pepper
tt	FiberMega

1. Boil potatoes, then drain excess water.
2. In a separate large stockpot, simmer mirepoix in water for 5 minutes.
3. Add all other ingredients and simmer for 10 minutes.
4. Season well and serve.

Southwestern Vegetables

1 can	tomato puree
1 can	black beans
1 lb.	frozen pepper/onion mix
½ lb.	frozen corn
4 oz.	frozen kale or collard greens
1 lb.	brown rice
1 tbsp.	chili powder
1 tsp.	cumin
tt	salt and pepper
tt	FiberMega

1. Cook brown rice in a separate pot.
2. Place all other ingredients in a large pot and simmer for 10 minutes.
3. Season to taste.
4. Serve over rice.

Stuffed Coconut Dates with Nut Butter

10 ea.	Medjool dates
10 tsp.	nut butter
½ cup	coconut, shredded

1. Carefully split Medjool dates in half and remove pits.
2. Fill each half with 1 teaspoon nut butter.
3. Sprinkle with coconut.

Note: you can use any type of nut butter, such as almond, cashew, hazelnut, macadamia, peanut, pecan, pistachio, or walnut.

Tomato Sauce

1 can	tomatoes, crushed, 28 oz.
1 can	tomato paste, 6 oz.
4 oz.	onions (fresh or frozen)
1 clove	garlic, minced
tt	basil, dried or fresh
tt	salt and pepper
tt	FiberMega

1. Place all ingredients in a saucepan and simmer.
2. Taste, season, and serve.

Pasta Primavera

1 lb.	pasta, whole wheat
1 can	tomatoes, diced, 28 oz.
1 can	kidney beans
1 lb.	frozen mixed vegetables
4 oz.	frozen kale or collard greens
1 lb.	water
tt	Italian spice mix
tt	salt and pepper
tt	FiberMega

1. Cook whole-grain pasta in a separate pot.
2. When pasta is done, place all ingredients in a large pot and simmer for 10 minutes.

Note: you can use any shape of pasta for this. Done is when the food smooth to the bite and has no crunch or hardness to the bite.

Banana Berry Smoothie

1 cup	water
2 ea.	Medjool dates, diced
1 ea.	banana, frozen
1 cup	frozen berry mix
1 tbsp.	FiberMega

1. Place water, bananas, and dates in blender and blend.
2. Add berries and FiberMega, then blend again.
3. Serve.

Chocolate Berry Smoothie
2 tbsp.	cocoa powder
1 ea.	diced frozen mango
1 tbsp.	FiberMega

1. Place mango in food processor and blend until smooth.
2. Add cocoa powder and FiberMega and blend until smooth.
3. Serve.

Note: you can substitute two very ripe frozen bananas for the mango.

Kale Smoothie
1 cup	water
2 ea.	Medjool dates, diced
½ bunch	kale, fresh
1 ea.	lemon, fresh
tt	cinnamon, ground
1 tbsp.	FiberMega

1. Place water, dates, lemon, and kale in blender and blend.
2. Add cinnamon and FiberMega and blend until smooth.
3. Serve.

Organic Food: Is It Worth the Price?

Organic farmers, ranchers, and food processors follow a defined set of standards to produce organic food and fiber. Congress described general organic principles in the Organic Foods Production Act, and the USDA defines specific organic standards. These standards cover the product from farm to table, including soil and water quality, pest control, livestock practices, and rules for food additives.[1]

It is my belief that most people buy organic food because they think it is more nutritious than conventional food—an assumption with which I disagree. Based on the definition of organic food, there is nothing different about its nutrients. When you compare conventional food to organic food, the bottom line is that conventional food has toxins, and organic food does not have toxins (or at least doesn't have as many).

According to Dr. Michael Greger, the author of *How Not to Die*, "Conventional produce appears to have twice the levels of cadmium, one of the three toxic heavy metals in the food supply, along with mercury and lead. The cadmium is thought to come from the phosphate fertilizers that are added to conventional crops."[2]

Many opponents of organic foods believe organic foods cost more than regular food, and I agree they do. I have seen this at the markets where I shop. In my opinion, the cost-benefit of a healthier body later in life is worth a few dollars spent today. The bottom line is that it is up to you.

Notes

[1] "USDA Organic|USDA." 2016. United States Department of Agriculture. Accessed May 17, 2016. http://www.usda.gov/wps/portal/usda/usdahome?navid=organic-agriculture/.

[2] Greger, M., and G. Stone. 2015. *How Not to Die: Discover the Foods Scientifically Proven to Prevent and Reverse Disease.* New York, NY: Flatiron Books.

CHAPTER 7
Summary

Now that you understand the meaning of Empty Eating and the reasons people gain weight and have unhealthy bodies, let's look at some background information about overeating and empty calories. Because I've introduced you to intermittent fasting already, we can begin to discuss strategies for losing that extra weight, as well as for developing a plan to achieve optimal health and wellness.

Before I offer suggestions for changing your health and lifestyle, I would like to share my personal thoughts with you. I draw my recommendations from my own knowledge, the available science, and my professional experience. I would never recommend something I had not tried myself, that isn't doable, or that isn't good for you.

Numerous products in the health marketplace—such as diet plans, expensive equipment, and "magic" pills—promise weight loss and a fit body. The media is always bombarding the airwaves with propaganda and false promises that usually produce disappointment. Although some methods work, the success is often temporary. Let's focus on some key approaches to achieving overall well-being and a healthy body.

My research has revealed seven fundamental principles for successful weight loss and better health:

- The will to change
- Discipline
- Ongoing education
- A healthy social relationship with family and friends
- Daily physical activities
- Eating a plant-based diet
- Plenty of sleep

Personal effort is also required to make these changes. Remember this phrase: "No pain, no gain." There's a lot of truth to it.

Scientific research and personal experience have tested and proven the ideas I have presented in this book; however, some ideas and techniques are easier to apply for some people than they are for others. All of us are different. What works for me may not work for you, and vice versa, but the general plan I recommend will work for anyone.

The differences among us do not cancel the power of these principles. If I walk five miles a day to maintain my health, you may need to walk only three miles to achieve your physical goals. The point is that we all need daily physical activity.

The methods I propose in this book are both safe and proven successful. I guarantee your success if you start today. I promise your body will take care of you if you take care of your body. As Dr. Michael Klaper has stated, "Your body is always talking to you." It is up to you to start listening. As soon as you start a whole-food, plant-based lifestyle, your body will begin to heal itself. Within a short time, you will see and feel the overall positive results. You will have no need to diet and count calories if you maintain the seven essential principles listed above. With them, you will gain a body that is full of energy.

Allow me to provide guidelines for you to follow. You must develop your own detailed plan and stick with it, understanding that you may need to tweak it from time to time. Tweaking your program often means making small changes to help you stay on track toward your goals.

As an example, I have shown friends how to make smoothies using my recipe. When I check back in a week or two, they are still making smoothies, but they have made some adjustments. Instead of using one apple and a teaspoon of cinnamon, they now use two apples and a tablespoon of cinnamon. It is not a big change, but that change is more suited to that individual.

I am helping you build a foundation by teaching you how to change your lifestyle with positive choices that are good for your health, but the responsibility still rests on your shoulders. For any "stay healthy" system to be effective, it must not target just one aspect of healthy living.

Regulating your diet without changes to your physical activities will be much less effective than a balanced program will. The same will be true if you add more exercise without making the proper nutritional changes.

The best systems target mild changes in several aspects of your life, instead of extreme changes to just one part. Milder changes, with no strict guidelines, are much easier to begin and follow. A lack of discipline could cause you to give up after only a few days or weeks. The goal is to make long-lasting, positive changes in your life. According to Charles Duhigg, the author of *The Power of Habit*, the best way to break a bad habit is to replace it with a good habit.

I've based the system I use to keep healthy and lean on the concepts included in the previous chapters. It is a combination of a form of intermittent fasting, whole plant–based foods, and exercise.

I practice intermittent fasting by eating only between noon and 8:00 p.m. I eat mostly whole plant–based foods, so vegetables, fruits, nuts, and seeds make up most of my diet. I do not practice any form of restrictive diets or count calories. The only supplements I take are vitamins B12 and D, and I get my omega-3 fats from ground flax seeds by eating FiberMega with every meal.

I exercise daily. I prefer to ride my bike and walk, but running or doing light cardio exercise is also acceptable. I do not take any medication, and I am not overweight. I consider myself a healthy and happy person. I base my recommendations on my experiences and on scientific facts. In this chapter, I give examples from my life experiences to explain how to improve yours.

As noted in chapter 4, intermittent fasting takes many forms that are useful for different people's individual needs. Because I eat within an eight-hour window each day, I get sixteen hours of fasting, with half of it being rest and sleep. I find this method efficient, because I can easily avoid eating a few hours before and after I sleep. During those brief periods, my hunger levels are lower than they are during the day.

Of course, it is up to each person to decide on the method that works best for him or her. It may depend on your schedule and goals; for instance, the Leangains approach may be more useful for someone going to the gym and trying to build muscle and lose fat. Find the method that works best for you, and fit into your daily schedule and eating habits.

You must avoid overeating if you want to achieve the healthiest body possible. Overeating causes adverse effects that will keep you from maintaining a robust and lean body. Overeating comes in several forms and with varied side effects, but the results are usually the same—weight gain, emotional distress, and undesirable metabolic changes are inevitable with overeating. You should pay attention to everything you eat and accept responsibility for every calorie you put into your body.

Snacks, a sweet here and there, one or two meals too many, and fast food on the road all contribute to weight gain, because they contain empty calories. Most people typically consume empty calories from simple carbohydrates such as candy and doughnuts.

You can find carbohydrates in a broad range of both healthy and unhealthy foods. They come in a variety of forms, such as sugars and starch. Carbohydrates provide glucose, which the body converts to energy that's used to support physical activity and body functions.

Carbohydrates should be the most important source of energy for your daily activity. The quantities and types of nutrients in carbohydrate-based foods determine the quality of those foods. Foods that contain only simple sugars are almost never considered healthy, because they include so many empty calories that contribute to weight gain and increased blood sugar. You should never follow a diet plan that suggests you eliminate a whole category of food such as carbohydrates.

We should also consider fiber when talking about the role of carbohydrates in our diets, because fiber influences how we digest carbohydrates. It has multiple effects on the intestines and digestion, and healthy amounts of fiber can bind and reduce the volume of carbohydrates absorbed during a given period, making it easier for the body to process them.

Unhealthier sources of carbohydrates include white bread, pastries, sodas, candy, and other highly processed or refined foods, as well as foods that have had sugars added to them, such as some fast foods. These items contain easily digested carbohydrates that contribute to weight gain, interfere with weight loss, and may promote diabetes and heart disease.

As much as possible, eliminate processed foods, because they contain concentrated amounts of sugar and fat—empty calories! Avoiding empty calories is a crucial decision to make, and in some cases, it will require you to give up sweet, highly processed foods that taste delicious but are not healthy for your body.

Exercise is another important factor contributing to overall health. You should select activities that support your unique goals. You may feel more comfortable jumping rope than you do swimming. As with various diets and fasting plans, different exercise programs give unique results. Resistance exercise, cardio exercise, yoga, strength training, and other forms of physical activity, regardless of their secondary goals (such as gaining muscle mass, losing weight, or improving the metabolism and blood flow), have one thing in common: they all benefit your general health and well-being.

You can consider exercise a pillar of good health. It increases blood flow, burns up excess calories, helps boost the immune system, optimizes metabolism, helps control blood sugar, and improves mood. Depending on the level of effort required, some workout programs can show benefits when practiced only a few days a week. I have found that exercising three to five days per week is usually optimal for showing results, although light exercise every day of the week is also a good option (e.g., I walk daily).

As I've mentioned, I usually walk, although riding my bike and using my treadmill are my backups. I do sit-ups and push-ups weekly. For some, riding a bike is a useful type of exercise; it can be effective when you want to cover distances that may be too far to walk. All these exercises can boost blood flow, improve cardiovascular health, and help burn off excess calories, and they offer the valuable benefit of being a second mode of transportation. Whatever activity you choose, make sure it's one you enjoy.

Combining your diet, a fasting method, and the right type of exercise is vital to achieving peak results.

A whole plant–based diet is the diet of choice for me. When I am eating whole plant–based foods, I get many benefits with little or no downside. Plant-based foods naturally contain fewer calories than animal-based foods do, and the plant-based food contains much more fiber (animal foods almost never include any); plus, plant-based food contains phytochemicals and a lot of vitamins and minerals. Plant-based protein is easier to digest and absorb than animal-based proteins are and contains the fiber and micronutrients needed to optimize the function of the digestive tract. That being said, animal-based foods are not "evil" per se—they are just being overconsumed in modern society and will lead to some complications if you eat them daily.

Plant-based foods contain no cholesterol and no bad fats, so they're better for you. Plant-based protein and carbohydrates make up most of my diet, and these are what I recommend for anyone trying to achieve peak physical health. That said, you might want to eat some animal-based foods occasionally; for example, once a week you may want to have some beef. Go for it. The problem is when you have that beef daily. A good guideline is to eat at least 85 percent whole plant–based foods.

When trying to better your health through nutrition, one of the most useful things to do is prepare your own meals. This is especially helpful if you practice a form of fasting, as you usually have fewer meals in a day.

The diet you choose should depend on your goals and your schedule. Breakfast can be made up of whole oats, dried fruits (especially berries), and some seeds and nuts. Lunch and dinner can include varieties of plant-based foods. Home-cooked items are the best, but vegan and vegetarian restaurants can provide healthy meals as well. In between meals, snacks such as fruits and/or smoothies may be a good choice; this way, you will always feel full, and you will be less likely to overeat. Nuts and seeds can also be excellent snacks in small amounts, both to obtain healthy fats and to help keep you full.

Most importantly, remember that you are solely responsible for what you eat and how you live your life. We live in an age with many choices and opportunities. Healthy foods are abundant...as are unhealthy ones. Educating yourself on what to eat is your—and only your—responsibility; it is necessary if you are to be fit and healthy.

—Chef Bill Collins

GLOSSARY

Adipose: Adipose refers to tissue made up mainly of fat cells, such as the yellow layer of fat beneath the skin.

Alzheimer's disease: A common form of dementia, doctors believe Alzheimer's disease is caused by changes in the brain, usually beginning in late middle age and characterized by memory lapses, confusion, emotional instability, and progressive loss of mental ability.

Angina: Caused by an inadequate blood supply to the heart, this condition causes severe pain in the chest and often spreads to the shoulders, arms, and neck.

Antibiotics: Medicines used to treat infections or diseases caused by bacteria, antibiotics work by blocking vital processes in bacteria, killing the bacteria or preventing them from multiplying. This helps the body's natural immune system to fight the bacterial infection.

Carbohydrates: These substances contain the glucose the body needs for energy. There are two main types of carbohydrates: simple and complex. The more refined or simple the carbohydrate, the more quickly it is converted to glucose and released into the bloodstream. This can cause peaks and dips in blood-sugar levels and result in varying energy levels.

Complex carbohydrates: These are sugars with complex molecular structures of three or more parts. Due to the complex structure of these molecules, it takes the body longer to break them down to produce the glucose it needs for energy. Foods rich in complex carbohydrates are green vegetables; whole grains and foods made from whole grains, such as oatmeal, pasta, and whole-grain bread; starchy vegetables, such as sweet potatoes, corn, and pumpkin; and beans, lentils, and peas.

Dementia: This refers to a chronic or persistent disorder of the mental processes caused by brain disease or injury and marked by memory disorders, personality changes, and impaired reasoning.

Fat: Oily solids or liquids in food, fats are an essential part of our diet and nutrition, and we cannot live without them. Our bodies require small amounts of "good fat" to function and to help prevent disease; however, many modern diets contain far more fat than the body needs. Too much fat, especially if it's the wrong type, can cause serious health complaints, including obesity, high blood pressure, and high cholesterol levels, which in turn lead to a greater risk of heart disease. There are two main types of fat: saturated and unsaturated. Doctors and dietitians generally consider unsaturated fats better for us than saturated fats are.

Fatty acids: These are the building blocks of the fat in our bodies and in the foods we eat. During digestion, the body breaks fats down into fatty acids, which then can be absorbed into the blood. Fatty acid molecules are usually joined in groups of three, forming a molecule called a *triglyceride*. Our bodies also make triglycerides from the car-bohydrates we eat.

Fatty acids have many important functions in the body, including energy storage. If glucose (a type of sugar) is not available for energy, the body uses fatty acids to fuel the cells instead.

Fiber: The indigestible part of plant food, also known as roughage, that pushes through our digestive system, absorbing water along the way and easing bowel movements. The word *fiber* comes from the Latin word *fibra*, meaning *thread, string, filament,* or *entrails.* Dietary fiber refers to nutrients in the diet that gastrointestinal enzymes don't digest.

Free radicals: Atoms or groups of atoms with an odd (unpaired) number of electrons, these can be formed when oxygen interacts with certain molecules. Once formed, these highly reactive radicals can start a chain reaction like dominoes. Their chief danger comes from the damage they can do when they react with important cellular components, such as DNA or the cell membrane (cells may function poorly or die if this occurs). To prevent free-radical damage, the body has a defense system of *antioxidants*.

Ghrelin: A hormone that increases appetite. Also known as *lenomorelin*, it is a peptide hormone produced by ghrelinergic cells in the gastrointestinal tract, which function as a neuropeptide in the central nervous system.

Glucose: Glucose is a carbohydrate and the most important simple sugar in human metabolism. Often called a simple sugar, or monosaccharide, because it is one of the smallest units with the characteristics of this class of carbohydrates, glucose is one of the primary molecules that serve as energy sources for plants and animals. You can find glucose in the sap of plants and in the human bloodstream, where we call it *blood sugar*.

Hormone: Produced in the body, this chemical controls and regulates the activity of certain cells or organs. Special glands, such as the thyroid, secrete the many hormones our bodies need. Hormones are essential for every activity of life, including the processes of digestion, metabolism, growth, reproduction, and mood control. Many hormones, such as neurotransmitters, are active in more than one physical process.

Insulin: A protein pancreatic hormone secreted by the beta cells of the islets of Langerhans that is essential, especially for the metabolism of carbohydrates and the regulation of glucose levels in the blood. Insufficient insulin production results in diabetes mellitus.

Ketone bodies: Acids made when the body starts using fat instead of carbohydrates for energy. When there is not enough insulin to get sugar from the blood and into the cells, the body turns to fat for energy. When fat is broken down, the body produces ketone bodies, which can accumulate in the body. High levels of ketones are toxic to the body, a condition called *ketoacidosis*.

Leptin: A hormone made by fat cells that decreases appetite, leptin is a *satiety hormone* produced by adipose cells. It helps to regulate energy balance by inhibiting hunger.

Metabolism: The rate at which the body's many processes function, it can be low, high, or somewhere in the middle. When we're young, our high metabolism makes it easy to lose weight. But as we get older, our metabolism slows down, and we might put on a few pounds. Exercising speeds up the metabolism.

Minerals: Minerals are inorganic elements that come from soil and water; they are absorbed by plants or eaten by animals. There are two kinds of minerals: *macrominerals* and *trace minerals*. The body needs larger amounts of macrominerals, such as calcium, phosphorus, magnesium, sodium, potassium, chloride, and sulfur, to grow and stay healthy; they assist in bone formation, hormone replenishment, and heartbeat regulation. We call other minerals, such as manganese, chromium, copper, iodine, iron, cobalt, fluoride, selenium, and zinc, trace minerals, because we only need minuscule amounts of them each day.

Neurodegenerative: Resulting in or characterized by degeneration of the nervous system, especially the neurons in the brain

Neurotropic factors: Molecules that enhance the growth and survival potential of neurons. They play important roles in both development, where they can act as guidance cues for developing neurons, and the mature nervous system, where they are involved in neuronal survival, synaptic plasticity, and the formation of long-lasting memories.

Parkinson's disease: This is a degenerative disorder of the central nervous system mainly affecting the motor system. Early in the course of the disease, the most obvious symptoms are movement related; these include shaking, rigidity, slowness of movement, and difficulty with walking and gait. Later, thinking and behavioral problems may arise, with dementia commonly occurring in the advanced stages of the disease, and depression being the most common psychiatric symptom.

Phytochemicals: A wide variety of compounds produced by plants, you can find these in fruits, vegetables, beans, grains, and other plants. Phytochemicals include antioxidants, flavonoids, phytonutrients, flavones, isoflavones, catechins, anthocyanidins, isothiocyanates, carotenoids, allyl sulfides, and polyphenols.

Proteins: These are large molecules consisting of amino acids. Without proteins, the body can't execute structural and functional regulation of body cells, tissues, and organs. Other forms of protein are enzymes, hormones, and antibodies. Proteins also work as neurotransmitters and carriers of oxygen in the blood (hemoglobin).

Pulmonary artery: This artery carries blood from the right ventricle of the heart to the lungs for oxygenation.

Pulmonary embolism: This is a blockage in one of the pulmonary arteries in the lungs. In most cases, pulmonary embolism is the result of blood clots that travel to the lungs from the legs or, rarely, other parts of the body (as in deep vein thrombosis).

Satiety: This is a feeling or condition of being full after eating food.

Vitamins: These are nutrients the body needs to maintain functions, such as immunity and metabolism. There are two types of vitamins: fat-soluble and water-soluble. When the body accumulates an excess of fat-soluble vitamins, they are stored in fat cells. Because they haven't been removed from the body, they are at some level of toxicity. They also need fat to be absorbed. Water-soluble vitamins are not stored in the body. The body takes what it needs from food and excretes what is not necessary as waste. It's easy to destroy water-soluble vitamins in foods during cooking, especially when high heat is applied. The answer is to cook on a moderate heat.

Water-soluble vitamins are thiamin (B1), riboflavin (B2), niacin (B3), B6, B12, biotin, folic acid (B9), pantothenic acid, and vitamin C. Fat-soluble vitamins are vitamin A, vitamin D, vitamin K, and vitamin E.

ABOUT THE AUTHOR

Chef Bill Collins
Phoenix, Arizona

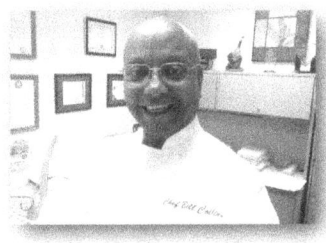

Chef Bill Collins grew up in Evansville, Indiana, and graduated from the prestigious Culinary Institute of America with his associate's and bachelor's degrees. He earned his master's degree from Northern Arizona University.

In recent years, Chef Bill became interested in a whole-food, plant-based diet lifestyle, because unhealthy eating is causing many illnesses that doctors cannot cure. Chef Bill is a published author, a culinary instructor, a culinary program director at Scottsdale Community College, a successful entrepreneur, and a person who believes in leading by example. Chef Bill eats what he dishes out. He believes overeating causes obesity, which is one of many reasons our society has so many obese and unhealthy people. Chef Bill says, "I want to help people change from eating the standard American diet to eating healthier, feeling better, and in the process dropping a few pounds. If you make a diet change and include some exercise, I guarantee you will become healthier and lose weight. I believe I can contribute to making your transition easier.

http://www.chefbillcollins.com
https://www.facebook.com/ChefBillCollins/
https://www.emptyeating.com
https://www.fibermega.com
https://www.facebook.com/fibermega/